Dermatology

IN*focus*

J D Wilkinson MB BS MRCS FRCP

Consultant Dermatologist, Amersham Hospital
Amersham, UK

S Shaw MB CHB FRCP

Honorary Consultant, Department of Dermatology
Amersham Hospital, Amersham, UK

D I Orton BSc MB BS MRCP

Consultant Dermatologist, Department of Dermatology
Amersham Hospital, Amersham, UK

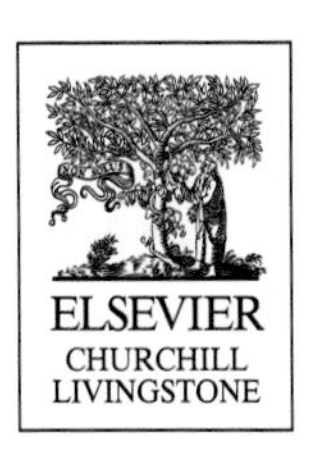

EDINBURGH LONDON NEW YORK OXFORD PHILADELPHIA ST LOUIS SYDNEY TORONTO 2005

ELSEVIER | CHURCHILL LIVINGSTONE
An imprint of Elsevier Limited

First published as Colour Aids—Dermatology 1987
First Colour Guide edition 1993
Second Colour Guide edition 1998
Reprinted 1999
Reprinted 2000
First In Focus edition 2005

ISBN 0443073767

British Library Cataloguing in Publication Data
A catalogue record for this book is available from the British Library

Library of Congress Cataloging in Publication Data
A catalog record for this book is available from the Library of Congress

Note
Medical knowledge is constantly changing. Standard safety precautions must be followed, but as new research and clinical experience broaden our knowledge, changes in treatment and drug therapy may become necessary or appropriate. Readers are advised to check the most current product information provided by the manufacturer of each drug to be administered to verify the recommended dose, the method and duration of administration, and contraindications. It is the responsibility of the practitioner, relying on experience and knowledge of the patient, to determine dosages and the best treatment for each individual patient. Neither the publisher nor the authors assumes any liability for any injury and/or damage to persons or property arising from this publication.

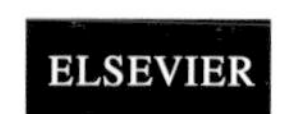

The publisher's policy is to use **paper manufactured from sustainable forests**

Printed in China

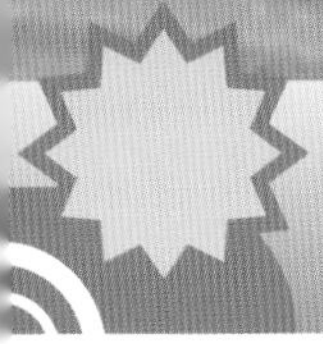

Acknowledgements

We would like to acknowledge the expert assistance of Alison Carter, Charles Day and Geraldine Thompson, Department of Medical Illustration, Wycombe and Amersham Hospitals. We also extend our thanks to the Department of Dermatology, The Churchill Hospital, Oxford, for their permission to reproduce illustrations borrowed from their collection. Fig. 203 was kindly provided by Dr Conlon, Genitourinary Medicine Physician at Oxford. The slide was taken by the Medical Illustration Department of the John Radcliffe Hospital. We also acknowledge the contribution made by Dr D A Fenton to the first edition of this book, and to Dr Graz Luzzi, Consultant Genitourinary physician, Wycombe General Hospital for help with the chapter on HIV/AIDS.

Amersham

J D W
S S
D O

Contents

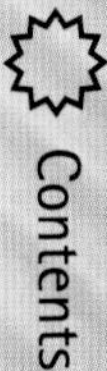

1 Benign childhood vascular tumours

Portwine stain (capillary haemangioma)

Aetiology

Developmental defect of mature dermal capillaries.

Clinical features

An erythematous or purplish macular naevus (Fig. 1) present at birth. It is usually unilateral, affecting face, trunk or limb, and variable in size. It may be associated with underlying arteriovenous malformation. Limb involvement may result in hypertrophy (Klippel–Trenaunay syndrome); a capillary naevus in the trigeminal area may be part of the Sturge–Weber syndrome.

Management

Cosmetic camouflage; argon or tuneable dye laser may help.

Strawberry naevus (cavernous haemangioma)

Aetiology

Developmental; benign angioblastic proliferation.

Clinical features

Develops rapidly during the first 6 months of life.
It is a well-demarcated, compressible vascular swelling (Figs 2 & 3) that normally undergoes spontaneous resolution. Haemorrhage, ulceration and thrombocytopenia are rare complications.

Management

None—spontaneous resolution. Surgery may be necessary for redundant folds of skin. High dose steroids are (rarely) given if severe thrombocytopenia, cardiac failure or vital functions, such as vision, breathing or feeding, are affected.

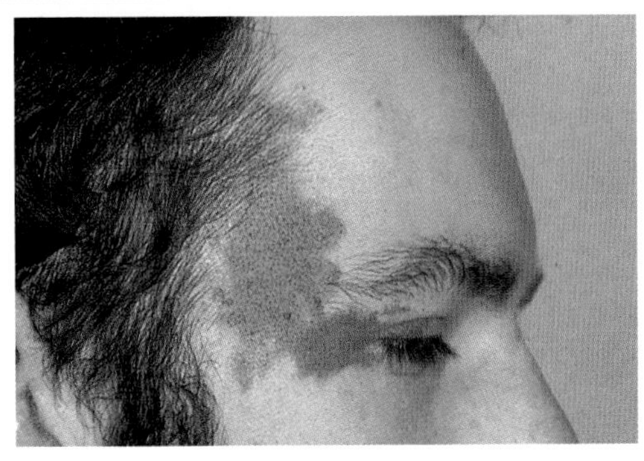

Fig. 1 Portwine stain.

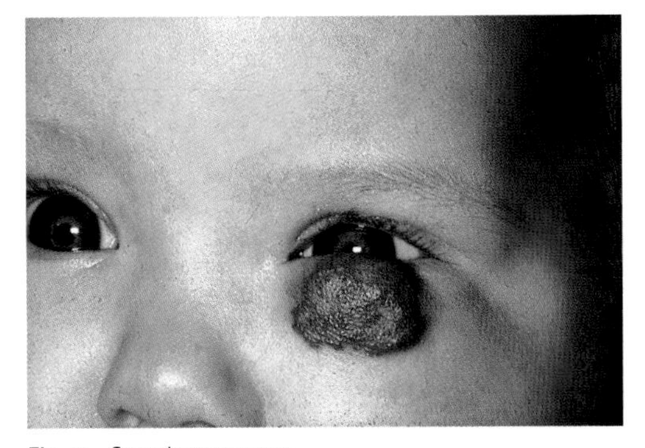

Fig. 2 Strawberry naevus.

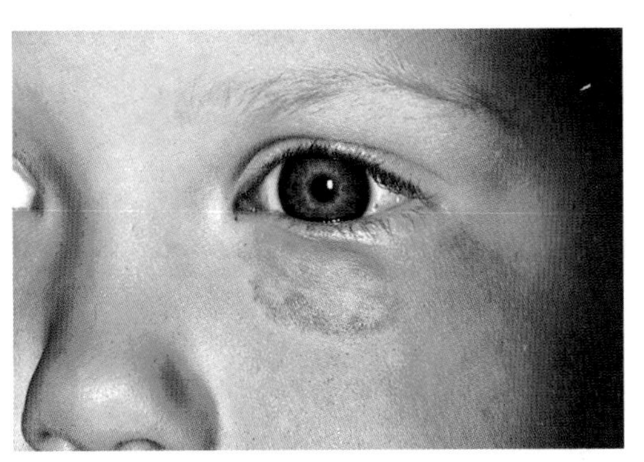

Fig. 3 Spontaneous resolution of same strawberry naevus.

Spider naevus

Aetiology

A small, superficial arteriole giving rise to a localized telangiectasia.

Clinical features

A central, raised, erythematous papule with radiating dilated capillaries. Lesions commonly occur on the face (Fig. 4) and often proliferate during pregnancy or liver disease. If lesions are multiple and involve mucosal surfaces, hereditary haemorrhagic telangiectasia should be considered.

Management

'Cold-point' cautery, vascular laser or 'epilating' electrodiathermy to the central arteriole. Some resolve spontaneously.

Lymphangioma circumscriptum

Aetiology

Localized lymphatic abnormality.

Clinical features

Fluctuating 'frog spawn-like' haemorrhagic vesicles (Fig. 5). Commonly presents in childhood.

Salmon patch

Aetiology

A localized, capillary, telangiectatic naevus.

Clinical features

A pale pink area, commonly found in newborn infants on the nape of the neck, on the glabella or over one eye (Fig. 6). No treatment is required.

Pyogenic granuloma

Aetiology

Abnormal proliferation of capillaries occurring after trauma or infection.

Clinical features

A friable and often pedunculated vascular nodule (Fig. 7), bleeding easily and profusely when traumatized.

Management

Curettage and cautery or excision under local anaesthetic. In adults, histology is necessary since the lesion can be confused with amelanotic malignant melanoma.

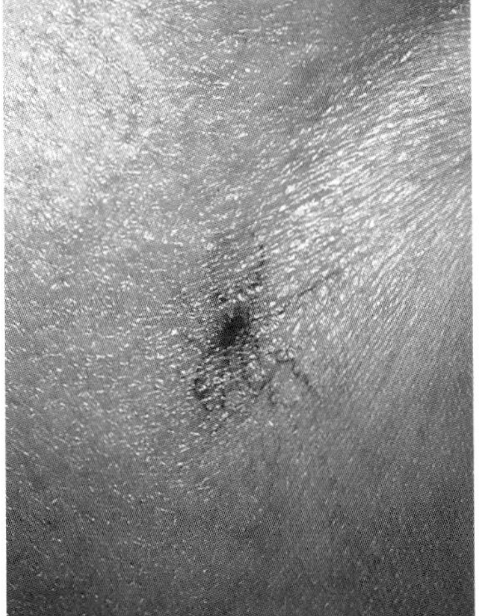

Fig. 4 Spider naevus.

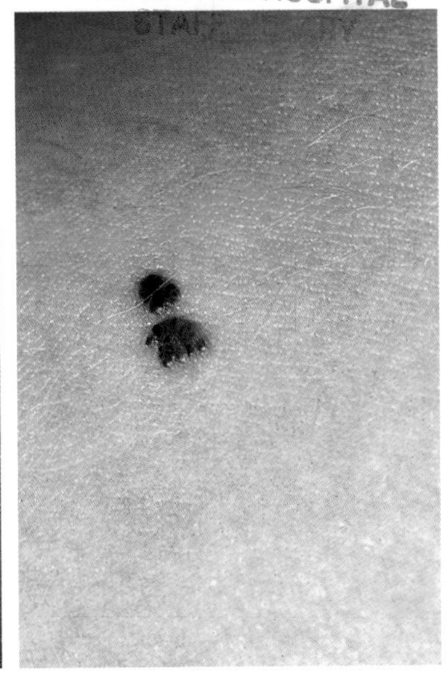

Fig. 5 Lymphangioma circumscriptum.

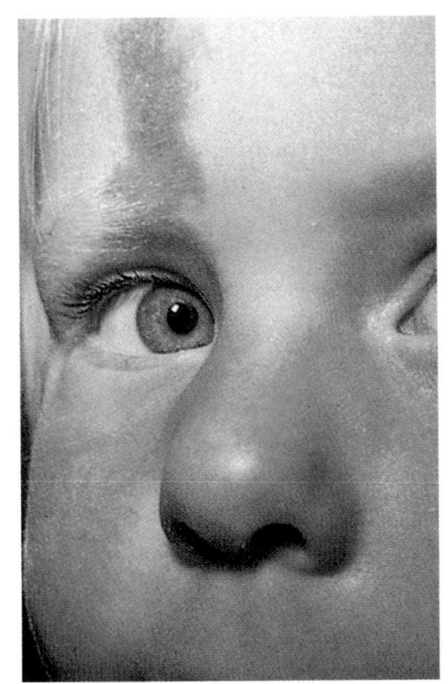

Fig. 6 Salmon patch. Facial lesions fade, but those on nape of neck may persist.

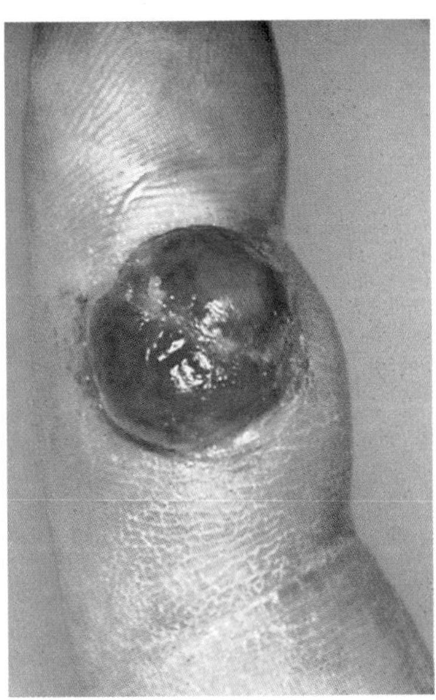

Fig. 7 Pyogenic granuloma. Grows rapidly, develops at sites of trauma.

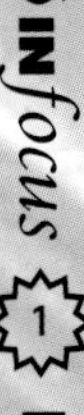

2 Benign childhood naevi

Freckles

Aetiology	Increased activity of melanocytes.
Clinical features	Brown macules (usually in redheads). They appear in early childhood and darken on sun exposure (Fig. 8).
Management	Sunscreens and sun protection.

Lentigo

Aetiology	A localized proliferation of melanocytes.
Clinical features	Areas of brown or black pigmentation, usually 1–2 mm in diameter. These appear in childhood but may proliferate in adulthood. They do not darken on sun exposure (Fig. 9).
Management	None. However, a solitary lentigo appearing in adult life or changing and growing may be a malignant melanoma.

Pigmented naevus/birthmark

Aetiology	Developmental defect.
Clinical features	Localized pigmented and sometimes hairy naevus (Fig. 10), present from birth, up to 2–3 cm in size. Giant hairy naevus is a rare developmental defect with a potential for malignant transformation. Surgical excision should be considered.
Management	None; excision if required.

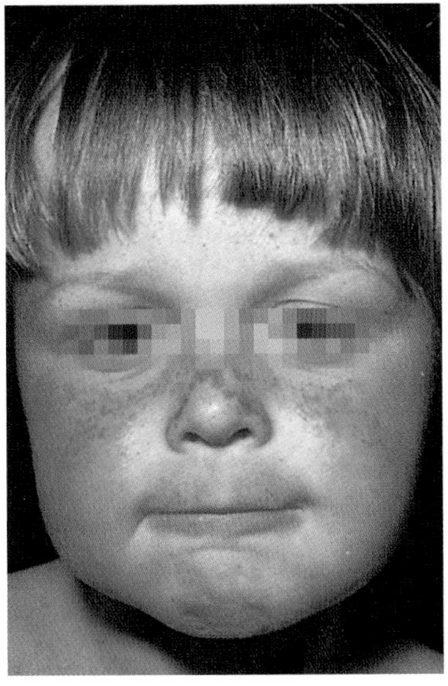

Fig. 8 Freckles.

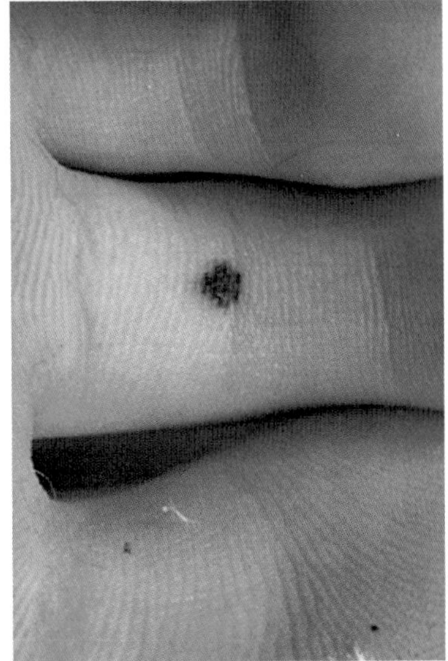

Fig. 9 Lentigo.

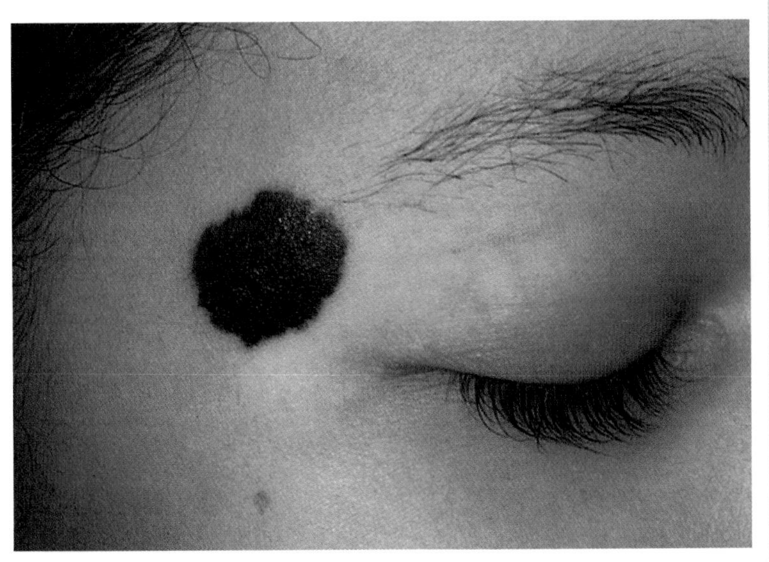

Fig. 10 Pigmented birthmark.

Cellular naevus

Synonym
Melanocytic or pigmented, compound or intradermal naevus.

Aetiology
Developmental defect. Melanocyte proliferation occurs at the dermo-epidermal junction or in the dermis.

Clinical features
Not normally present at birth, but develops during childhood and early adult life. It may be pink (Fig. 11), brown or black (Fig. 12), flat or raised, hairy or non-hairy. Blue naevus (Fig. 13) is a variant with dermal pigmentation. Malignant transformation is possible, especially in those with large numbers of 'atypical' pigmented naevi and a family history of melanoma. Some naevi develop surrounding hypopigmentation (halo naevi).

Management
Excision in cases of frequent trauma or should any individual mole change or darken in adult life. Excised moles should be submitted for histology.

Juvenile melanoma (benign)

Synonym
Spitz naevus.

Aetiology
A variant of cellular naevus.

Clinical features
A solitary, reddish-brown nodule occurring in childhood (usually affecting the face), growing rapidly to 1 cm. The lesion is benign, although the histology may resemble that of malignant melanoma (Fig. 14).

Management
None or simple excision.

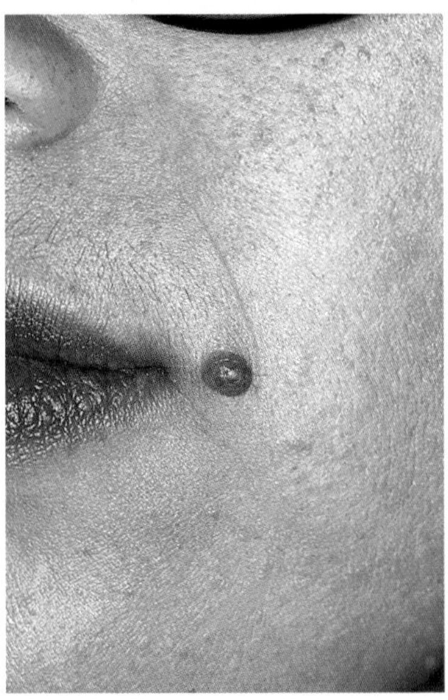

Fig. 11 Cellular or intradermal naevus.

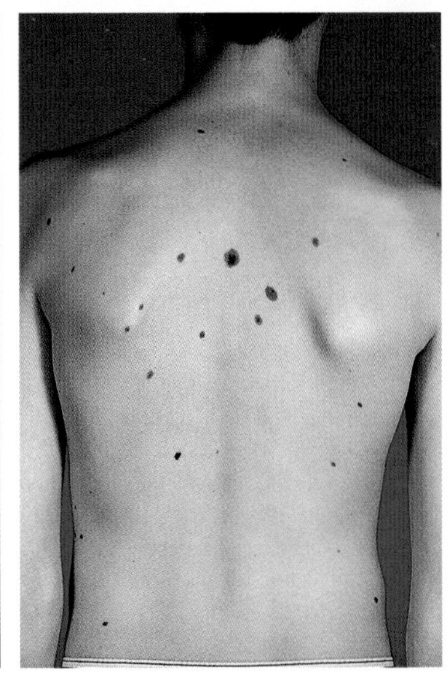

Fig. 12 Pigmented cellular naevi, some with surrounding hypopigmentation (halo naevus).

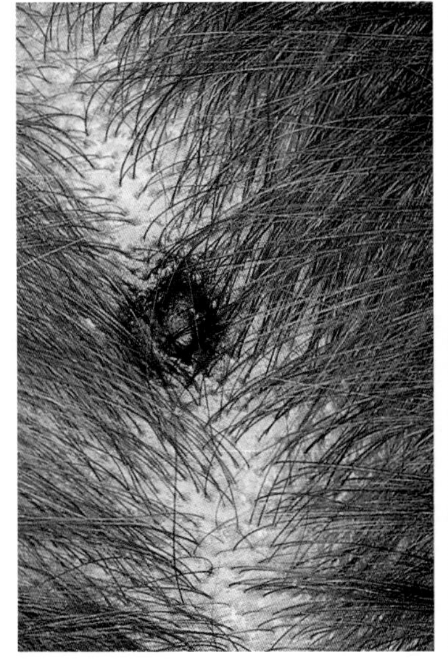

Fig. 13 Blue naevus.

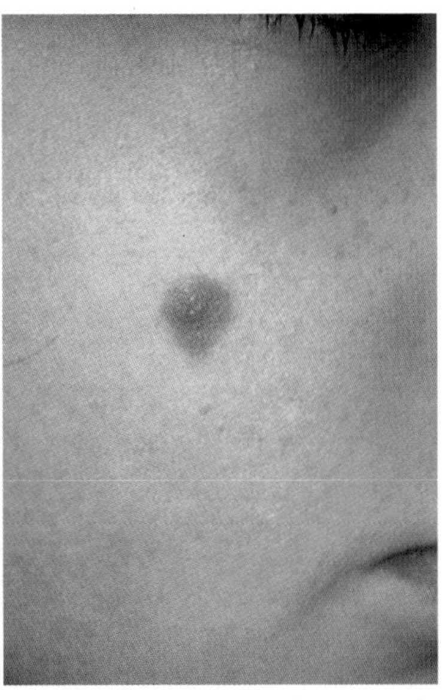

Fig. 14 Juvenile melanoma (Spitz naevus).

3 Napkin eruptions

Napkin candidiasis

Aetiology

Yeast infection with *Candida albicans*.

Clinical features

Well-demarcated erythema with scaling extending from the perineum, normally involving the skin folds. There may be isolated 'satellite' lesions with or without pustules. Oral lesions and intertriginous infections are common (Figs 15 & 16) (see also p. 120).

Management

Swabs; nystatin and imidazole creams (or a hydrocortisone/imidazole combination); reduction of occlusion and eradication of yeast carriage. An appropriate dusting powder may prevent relapse.

Napkin psoriasis

Aetiology

Local factors; possible genetic predisposition.

Clinical features

Develops suddenly, normally at about 4–8 weeks. Dark-red and scaly lesions with well-defined margins are seen in the napkin area (Fig. 17) and often on the scalp. Smaller scattered lesions can develop elsewhere on the trunk. Napkin area lesions are larger, are asymptomatic and may extend to the flexures. Often clears spontaneously within a few weeks.

Management

Bland applications and mild topical steroids or steroid plus antimicrobial combinations.

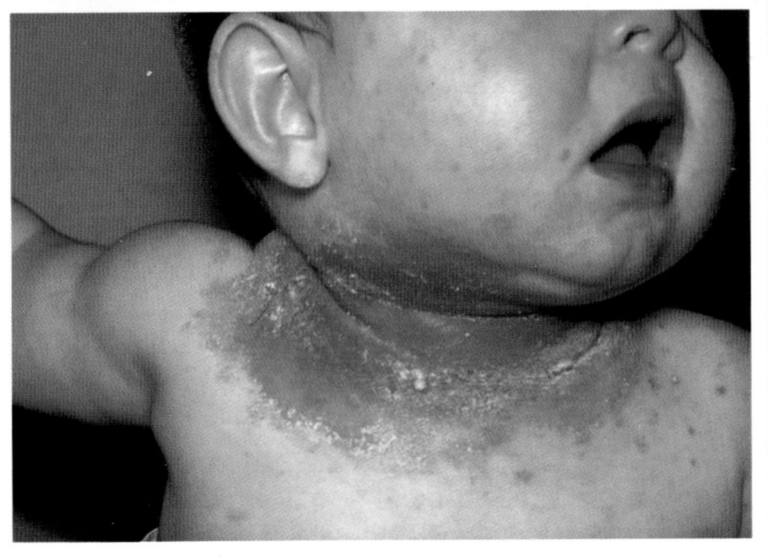

Fig. 15 Candidal intertrigo.

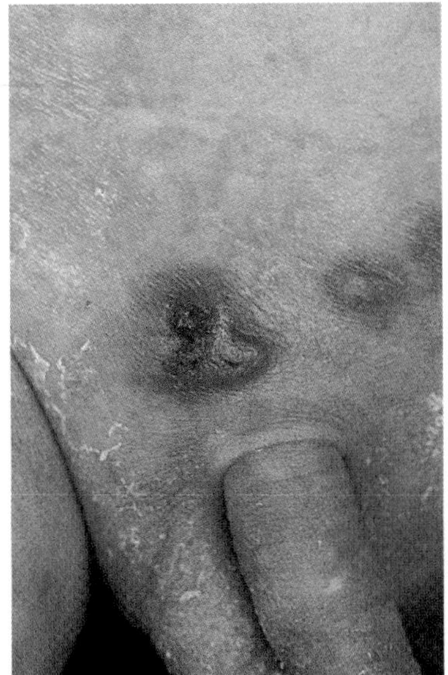

Fig. 16 Granuloma gluteale infantum (candida).

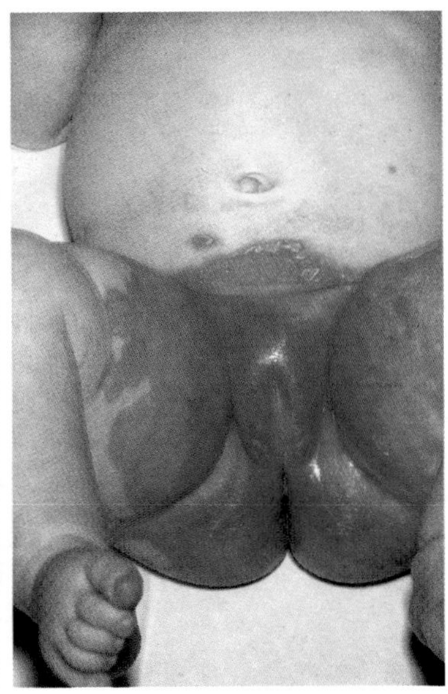

Fig. 17 Psoriasiform napkin rash.

Seborrhoeic eczema

Aetiology

Unknown. Constitutional and microbial factors may play a part. May be associated with atopy.

Clinical features

Appears at 2–10 weeks. Asymptomatic, well-defined, round or oval patches of erythema and greasy scaling extend to form gyrate patterns in the genitocrural flexures. Scalp, ears and other body folds may be involved (Fig. 18).

Management

Cleansing cream and mild topical steroid/imidazole.

Napkin dermatitis

Aetiology

Inflammatory disorder produced by prolonged contact with urine, faeces or irritant chemicals in napkin. It may be the first manifestation of atopic eczema.

Clinical features

Genitalia, buttocks, lower abdomen and upper thighs are affected. Flexures are normally spared (Fig. 19). Initial erythema, but vesicles, papules, erosions and ulcers may develop. Fine scaling with glazed erythema is seen in chronic forms.

Management

Emollients and weak topical steroid/antimicrobial. Frequent changing and thorough cleaning with a mild non-soap cleanser (e.g. aqueous cream). Plastic napkins or pants should be avoided and nappies left off where possible. A barrier cream can be used at night. Candidiasis or secondary bacterial infections should be treated appropriately.

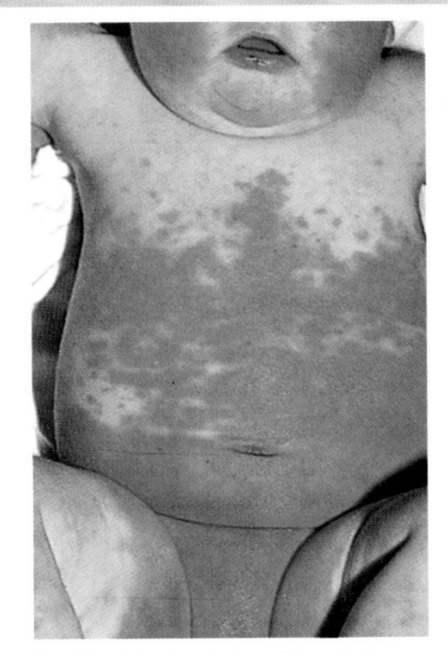

Fig. 18 Seborrhoeic dermatitis of infants.

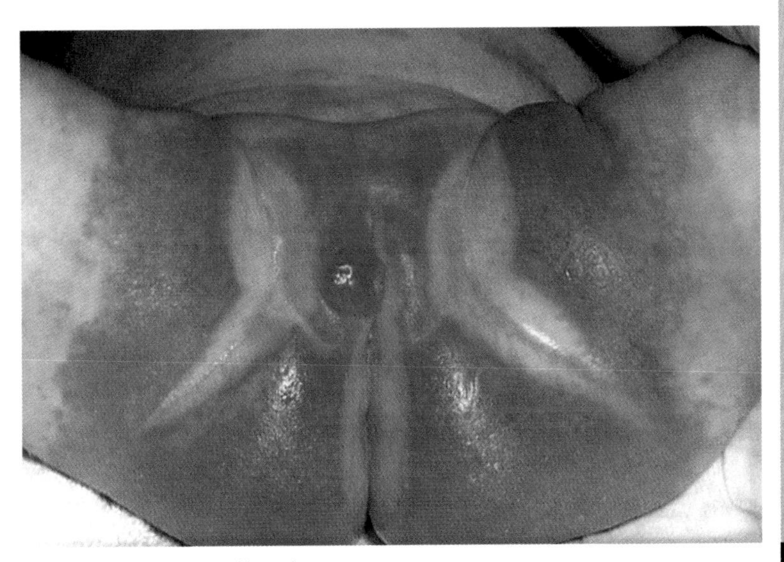

Fig. 19 Ammoniacal napkin rash.

4 Childhood scalp conditions

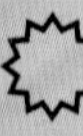

Cradle cap (seborrhoeic eczema)

Aetiology

Unknown; possible constitutional and microbial factors.

Clinical features

Appears at 0–3 months. The scalp is covered with 'greasy' scales (Fig. 20). The cheeks, flexures of neck, axillae, napkin areas and ears are often affected. It may mimic psoriasis.

Management

Oil or mild keratolytics (e.g. 2% salicylic acid in oil for the scalp); non-soap cleansers and hydrocortisone-imidazole combinations elsewhere.

Tinea/pityriasis amiantacea

Aetiology

Distinctive reaction pattern of scalp. It may be associated with psoriasis or eczema.

Clinical features

Asbestos-like, silvery scales adhere firmly to scalp and hair (Fig. 21). If associated infection is present, the underlying scalp is erythematous and moist. There may be some loss of hair.

Management

2% salicylic acid in oil or aqueous cream, tar-containing keratolytic preparations such as Ung. Cocois Co. with tar shampoos and steroid or steroid/antibacterial creams or gels. Occasionally systemic antibiotics and stronger tar or keratolytic preparations may be needed.

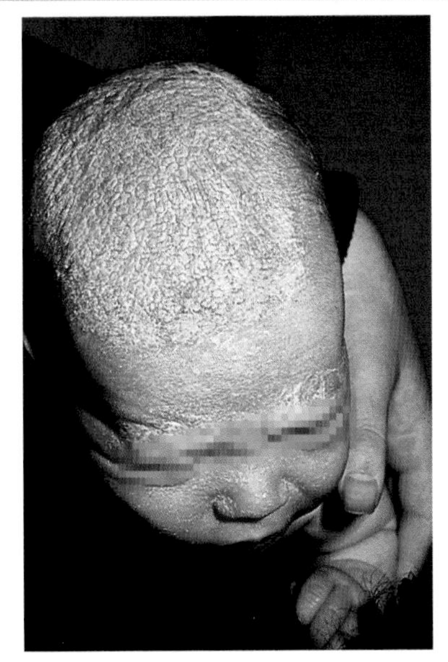

Fig. 20 Cradle cap.

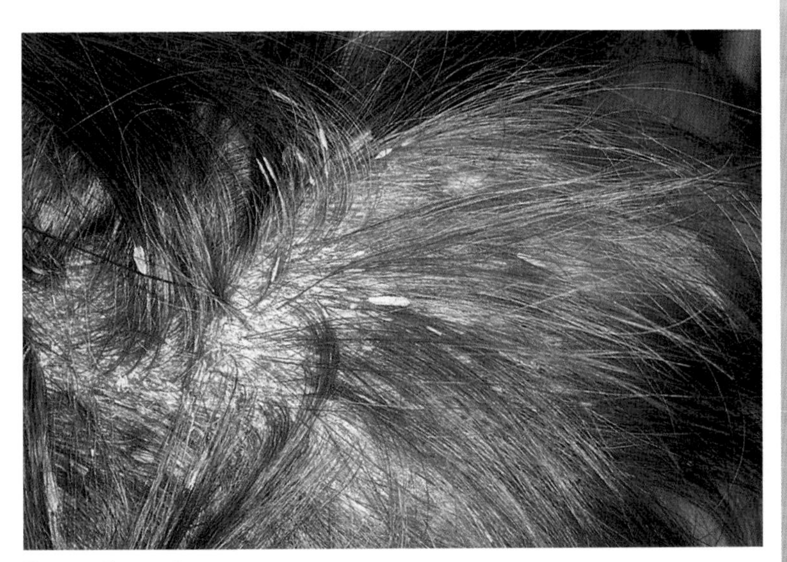

Fig. 21 Tinea amiantacea.

Ringworm

Synonym

Tinea capitis.

Aetiology

Microsporum audouinii and *M. canis* invade hair shafts. The former condition is now, fortunately, a rarity. *M. canis* is, however, commonly contracted from cats and dogs (especially puppies). *Trichophyton tonsurans* infection is endemic in some countries and is now a common cause of ringworm in urban areas. Animal trichophyton infections cause more severe reactions.

Clinical features

The condition is usually seen in children and produces circular, erythematous bald patches with scaling and broken hair shafts (Fig. 22). Wood's light examination shows a green or blue fluorescence for *M. audouinii* or *M. canis* (Fig. 23) but not for other types of fungus. A more inflammatory reaction follows infection with animal ringworm (cows, horses, etc.) (Fig. 24). This produces a tender and much more pustular kerion (Fig. 25), which may ultimately cause scarring alopecia. Fungal microscopy and culture are usually positive, but false-negative results may occur with kerion.

Management

Oral griseofulvin is still the treatment of choice in children. The affected hair should be cropped short and treatment continued for at least 6 weeks. Topical antifungal agents may also be used. Several newer oral antifungal drugs are now available for use in adults (e.g. terbinafine).

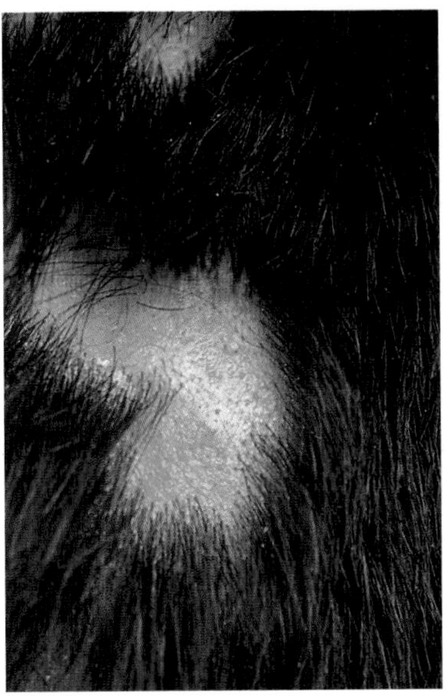

Fig. 22 Tinea capitis (microsporum).

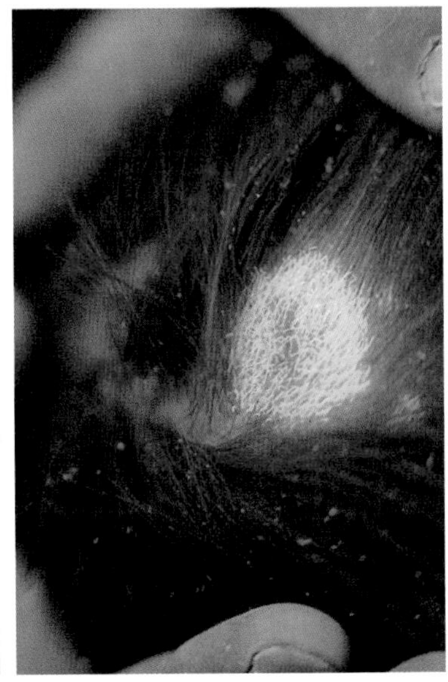

Fig. 23 Characteristic green-blue fluorescence under Wood's light.

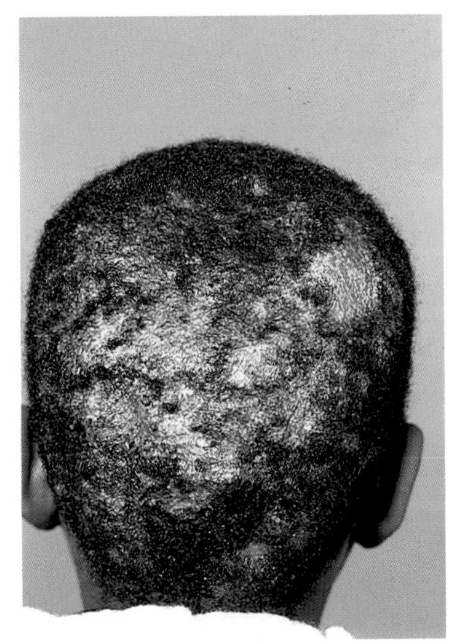

Fig. 24 Cattle ringworm.

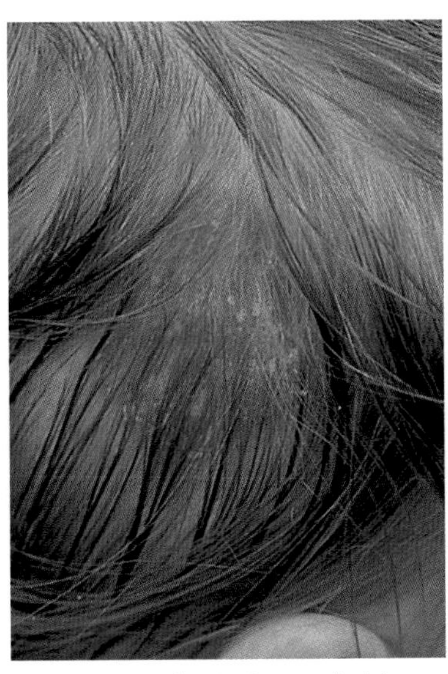

Fig. 25 Kerion (cattle ringworm) of the scalp.

5 Childhood bacterial infections

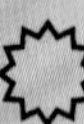

Impetigo

Aetiology

A contagious superficial skin infection caused by *Staphylococcus aureus* or group A β-haemolytic streptococci, or both.

Clinical features

Bullae may rupture to produce golden-yellow crusts (Fig. 26). The disease can become epidemic in overcrowded conditions. Scabies, lice and eczema predispose. Glomerulonephritis (streptococcus) and toxic epidermal necrolysis (staphylococcus) are rare complications.

Management

Swabs followed by topical or systemic antibiotics. Staphylococcal or streptococcal carriage should be eradicated from nose (staphylococci), throat (streptococci) and perineum (both) (Fig. 27). Close family members should be screened.

Infantile toxic epidermal necrolysis

Aetiology

Staphylococci (usually phage type 71) liberate toxins, leading to large superficial erosions. Drugs may produce a similar syndrome in adults.

Clinical features

A rare disease occurring after minor skin infections or impetigo in infants. The process mimics a burn or scald (Fig. 28). Untreated, the disease may be fatal.

Management

Swabs followed by appropriate systemic antibiotic therapy. Dehydration and electrolyte imbalance should be corrected. Treat topically, as for burns.

Toxic shock syndrome

Aetiology

Toxin produced by phage group I (usually penicillin-resistant) staphylococcal infection.

Clinical features

Fever, diarrhoea, shock and erythematous rash.

Management

General supportive measures. Penicillinase-resistant antibiotic therapy.

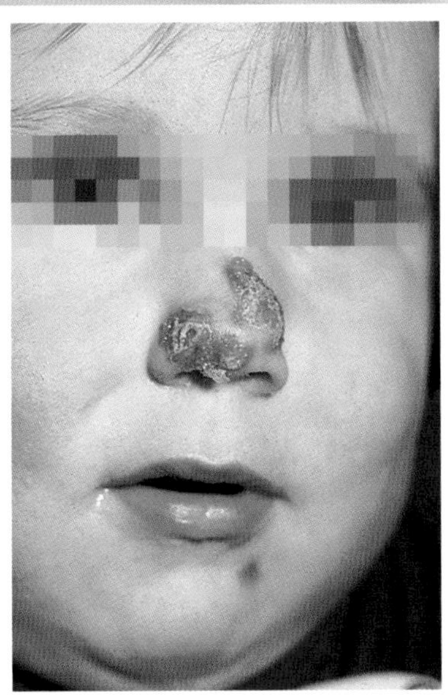

Fig. 26 Impetigo. Face and perioral region are frequently affected.

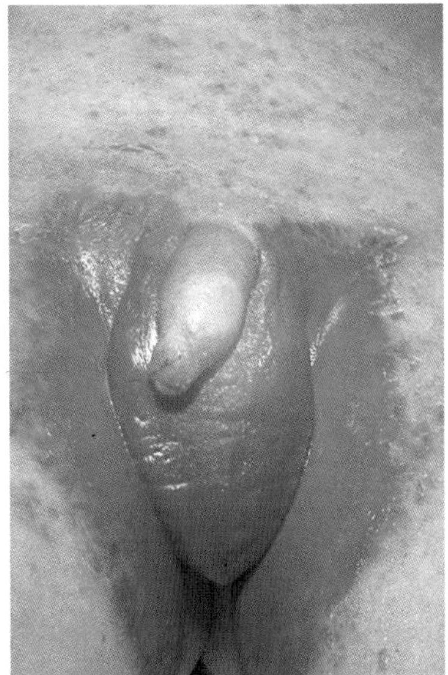

Fig. 27 Mixed staphylococcal and streptococcal intertrigo.

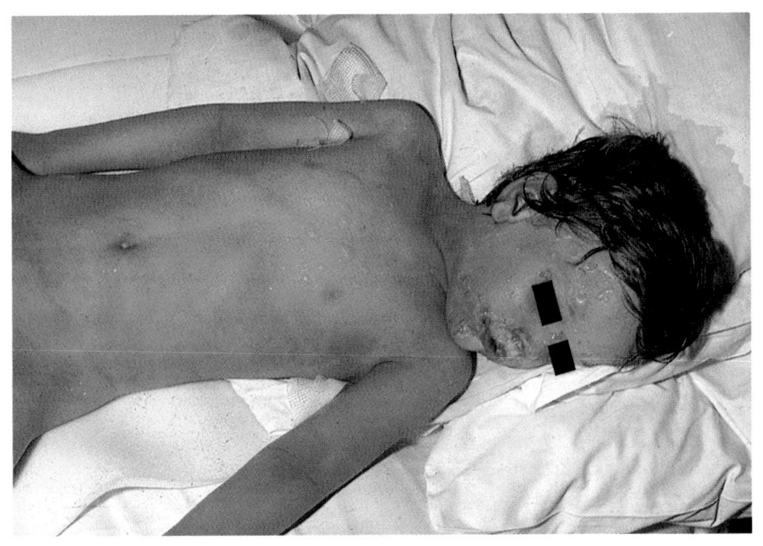

Fig. 28 Toxic epidermal necrolysis.

Warts

Aetiology

Reactive epidermal proliferation caused by infection with human papilloma virus.

Common wart

Clinical features

Elevated, hyperkeratotic papules with a rough surface occurring mainly on the hands (Fig. 29). They are solitary or multiple and arise in areas of trauma (especially the nail fold) (Fig. 30).

Treatment

Warts generally resolve spontaneously within 2 or 3 years. Treatment depends on type, number, site, age, patient's determination. Proprietary wart paints containing salicylic acid or glutaraldehyde combined with regular pumice and occlusion may be effective, as may freezing with liquid N_2, N_2O or CO_2 snow. (Several applications may be needed.) Rarely, curettage and cauterization are necessary.

Plantar warts (verrucae)

Clinical features

Deep, hyperkeratotic, often tender lesions on the sole (Fig. 31). They are differentiated from corns and calluses by paring; warts have areas of black speckling and fine bleeding points. Multiple superficial plantar warts may coalesce to form a 'mosaic wart', which is very resistant to therapy and implies poor natural resistance (Fig. 32).

Management

26%–50% salicylic acid paints or plasters or podophyllin/salicylic acid ointments combined with soaking, paring and occlusion or use of formaldehyde or glutaraldehyde solutions or intermittent treatment with liquid N_2. Therapy may be required for several weeks or months. Curettage and cautery may be employed for the occasional resistant verruca, but this treatment is painful. Immunotherapy, photodynamic therapy, intralesional bleomycin and laser treatment require specialist knowledge and expertise.

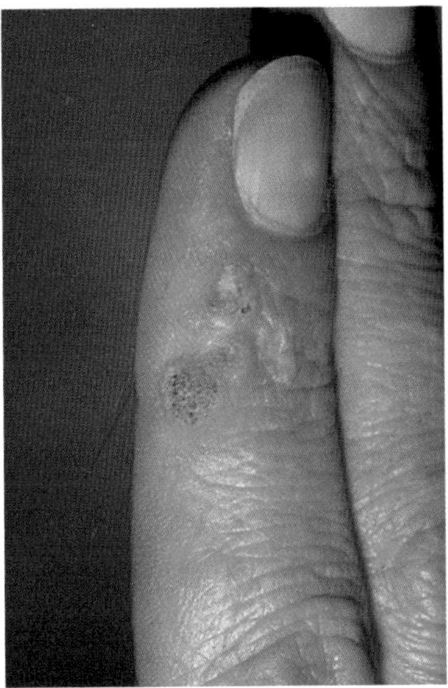

Fig. 29 Common warts.

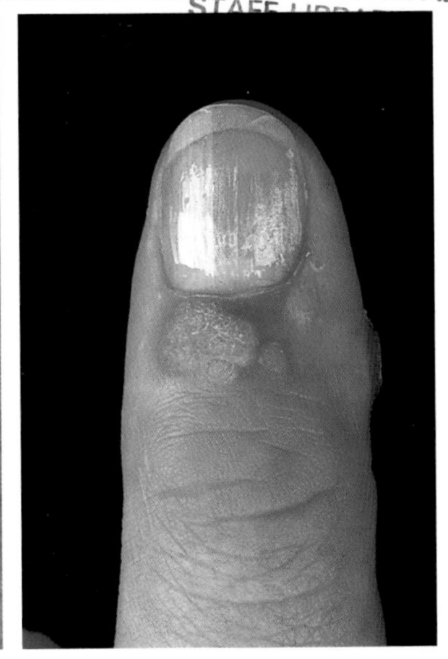

Fig. 30 Warts in nail fold.

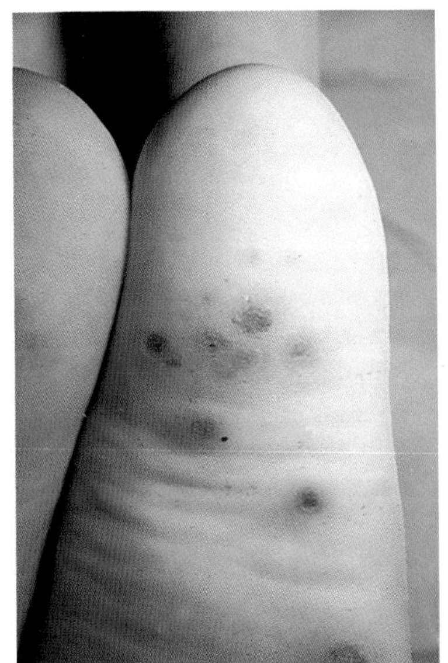

Fig. 31 Multiple plantar warts.

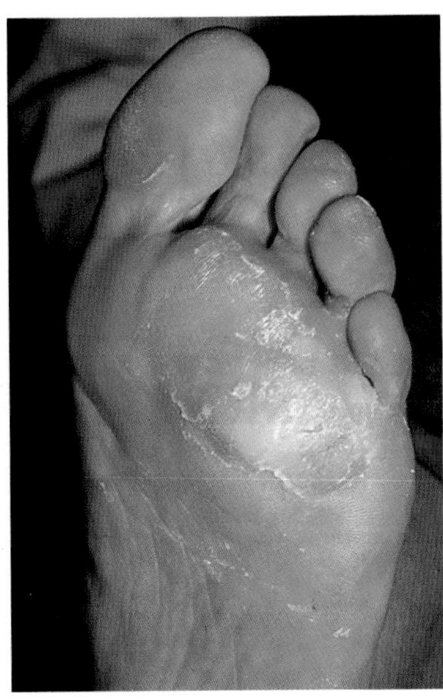

Fig. 32 Mosaic plantar wart.

Filiform warts

Clinical features

Small digitate warts that often appear in clusters on the Local anaesthetic creams can be applied prior to treatment if necessary.

Management

Cryotherapy, superficial cauterization or diathermy. Local anaesthetic creams can be applied prior to treatment if necessary.

Plane warts

Clinical features

Multiple smooth, small, flat-topped papules, which may be linear or coalesce due to trauma (Köbner phenomenon) (Fig. 34), occurring in young children and occasionally in adults. The face and backs of hands are particularly affected. They persist longer than other warts and respond less well to treatment. They will eventually disappear spontaneously.

Management

None (or placebo); tretinoin, 0.025%, or 5% 5-fluorouracil creams or light cryotherapy to induce mild to moderate irritation.

Genital warts (condyloma acuminata)

Aetiology

In children, infection may be associated with both genital and non-genital strains of human papilloma virus. Heteroinoculation and autoinoculation may both occur, and transmission may be both sexual and non-sexual.

Clinical features

Typically soft, pink, filiform or pedunculated lesions affecting the glans and prepuce (Fig. 35), vulva or perianal skin.

Management

Search for evidence of wart virus elsewhere. The possibility of sexual abuse and other sexually transmitted disease should be kept in mind. Treatment with intermittent topical imiquimod, 15–25% podophyllin, 0.5% podophyllotoxin with or without cryotherapy, 50–80% trichloracetic acid (NB: note contraindications and toxicity) or diathermy.

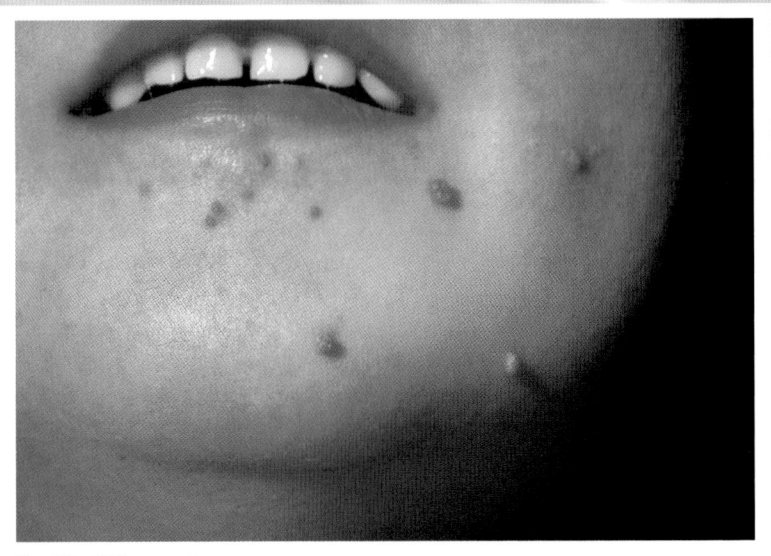

Fig. 33 Filiform warts.

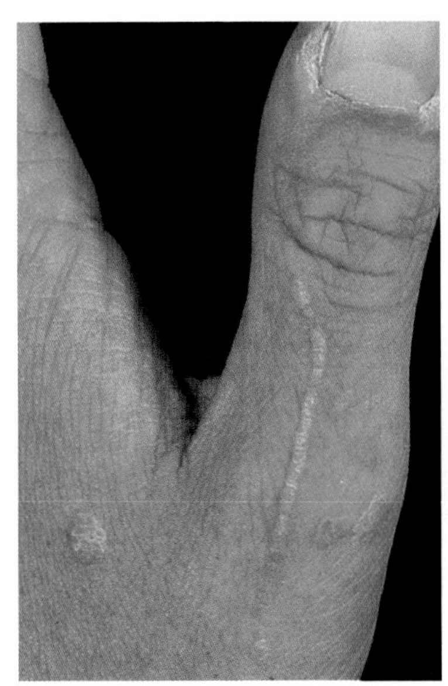

Fig. 34 Plane warts showing Köbner phenomenon.

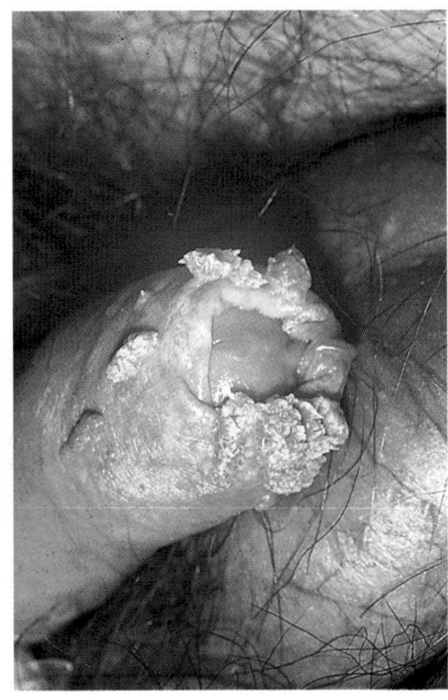

Fig. 35 Genital warts.

Molluscum contagiosum

Aetiology

Pox virus.

Clinical features

Common in childhood, especially in atopic persons. Lesions are characteristically grouped, pearly white or pink, firm, umbilicated papules (Fig. 36) with a central depression. Commonly affect the face, neck, trunk and perineum, although any area may be involved. They may grow to 5–10 mm in diameter if left untreated and soften as they mature. Some become inflamed, secondarily infected or eczematized.

Management

Lesions are easily treated with liquid nitrogen, may be 'spiked' with phenol or iodine, or painted with podophyllin. They can also be removed by curettage, diathermy or any other mildly traumatic procedure. Localized areas may be pre-treated with topical local anaesthetic and occlusion to facilitate treatment. Mollusca will, however, resolve spontaneously in time.

Hand, foot and mouth disease

Aetiology

Coxsackie virus infection; epidemic. It mainly affects young children.

Clinical features

The disease is usually mild, with an incubation period of 5–7 days. There are scattered vesicles in the mouth and on the palms or soles (Fig. 37). Those in the mouth soon break down to leave small ulcers (Fig. 38). In some children there may be a more widespread exanthem.

Management

None.

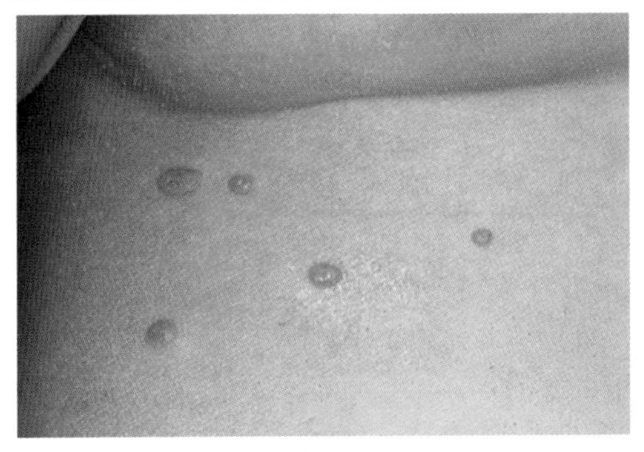

Fig. 36 Molluscum contagiosum.

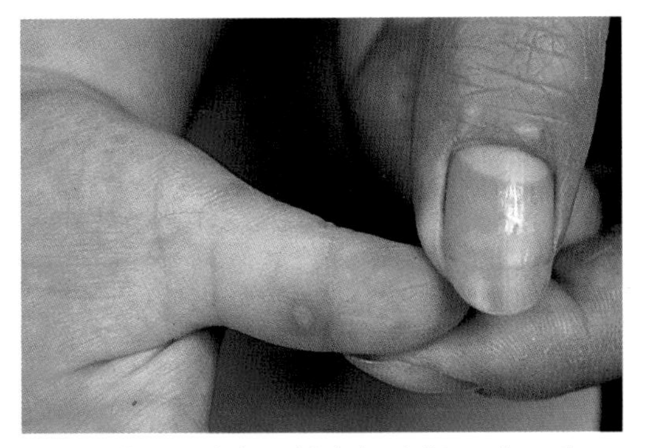

Fig. 37 Characteristic vesicle in hand, foot and mouth disease.

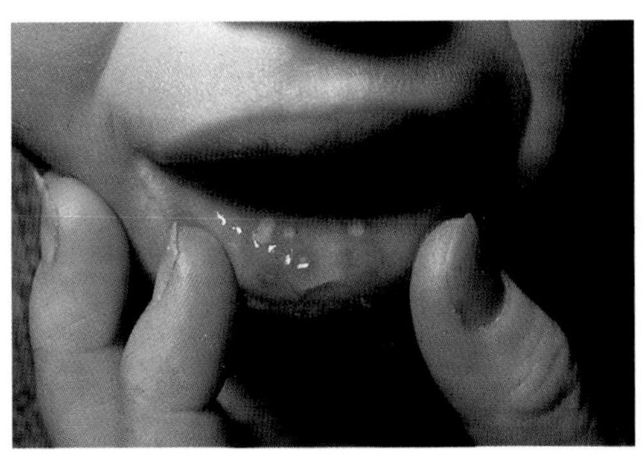

Fig. 38 Oral involvement in hand, foot and mouth disease.

7 Childhood infestations

Head lice (pediculosis capitis)

Aetiology

Common infestation in unhygienic or crowded conditions.

Clinical features

Severe pruritus, especially on the nape of neck and occiput. Lice may be present (Fig. 39), but nits (eggs) on hair shafts are diagnostic. Excoriations are common. Impetiginous secondary infection can occur. Exudation may cause matting of hair.

Management

Removal of nits with a fine-toothed metal comb. 1% permethrin or 0.5% carbaryl or malathion solution is applied to hair after washing. Repeated treatments may be necessary. Contacts must also be treated.

Insect bites (papular urticaria)

Aetiology

Hypersensitivity reaction to insect bites (e.g. fleas, bedbugs, mites).

Clinical features

Urticated papules occur in groups (Figs 40 & 41) and may be seasonal. Bullae can occur, particularly on the legs. Pruritus may be intense. Episodes may be recurrent or persist for several months. Impetigo can be a complication.

Management

Symptomatic. Treat the source if possible (including pets). Systemic antihistamines and topical steroids may be useful. See also Infestations (p. 122).

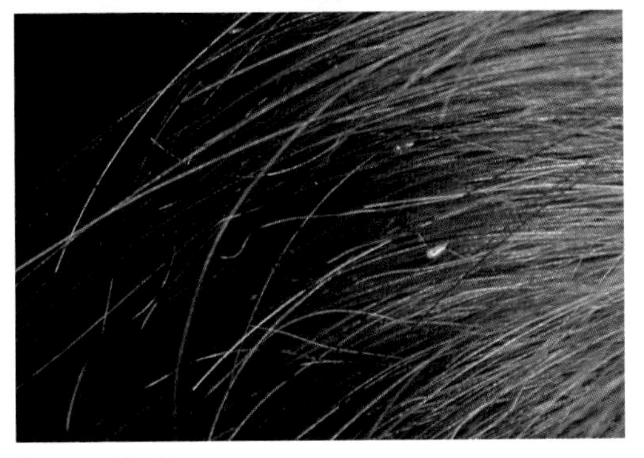

Fig. 39 Head louse.

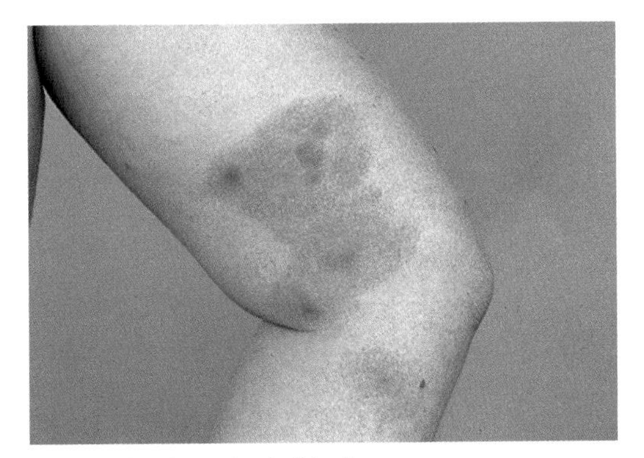

Fig. 40 Papular urticaria (bites).

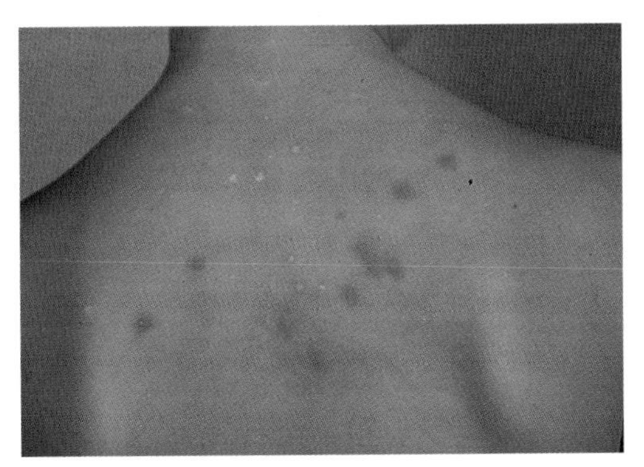

Fig. 41 Characteristic pattern of lesions as seen in insect bites.

8 Atopic eczema

Asthma, hay fever and infantile eczema tend to run in families. Up to 30% of the population are potentially 'atopic', although only 10% develop eczema.

Synonym

Infantile eczema.

Aetiology

Inheritance of atopic diathesis; sensitivity or allergy to foreign proteins (type I hypersensitivity reactions); a dry, sensitive, easily irritated and eczema-prone skin, aggravated by hard water, cold (low humidity), heat, sweating, woollen clothing, infections and stress.

Clinical features

Atopic eczema can occur at any age, but it often develops about 3 months after birth. Intense pruritus is a prominent feature (Fig. 42).

Facial The face is often involved in babies (Fig. 43). Itchy, erythematous papules on the cheeks or erythematosquamous dry ('chapped') or hypopigmented areas may be seen. Infraorbital lines (Morgan's folds) are common in atopic individuals. Constant licking of lips in some children causes 'lick eczema'.

Flexural Characteristic in early childhood. There is symmetrical involvement of elbow and knee flexures, wrists and ankles. The skin is generally dry and lichenified or excoriated.

Lichenification Constant rubbing and scratching gives rise to areas of thickened skin with increased skin markings. This is particularly seen around flexures (Fig. 44).

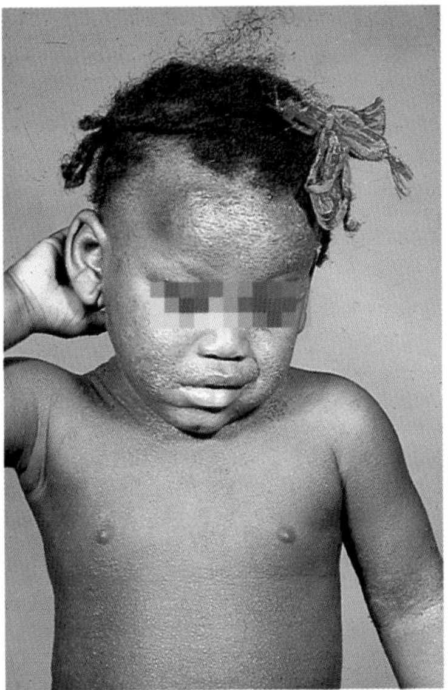

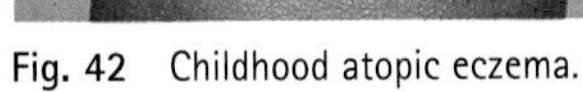

Fig. 42 Childhood atopic eczema.

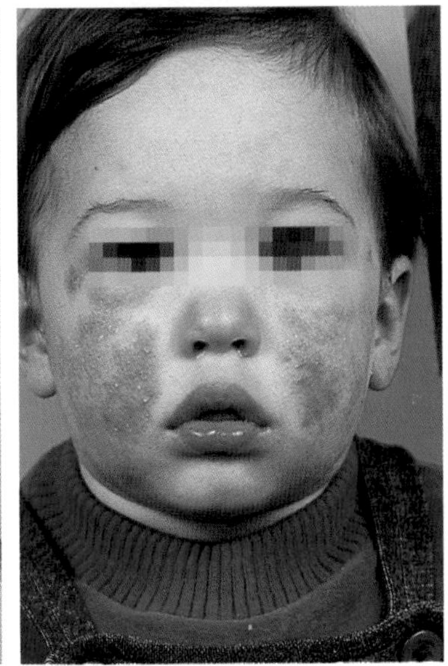

Fig. 43 Facial atopic eczema.

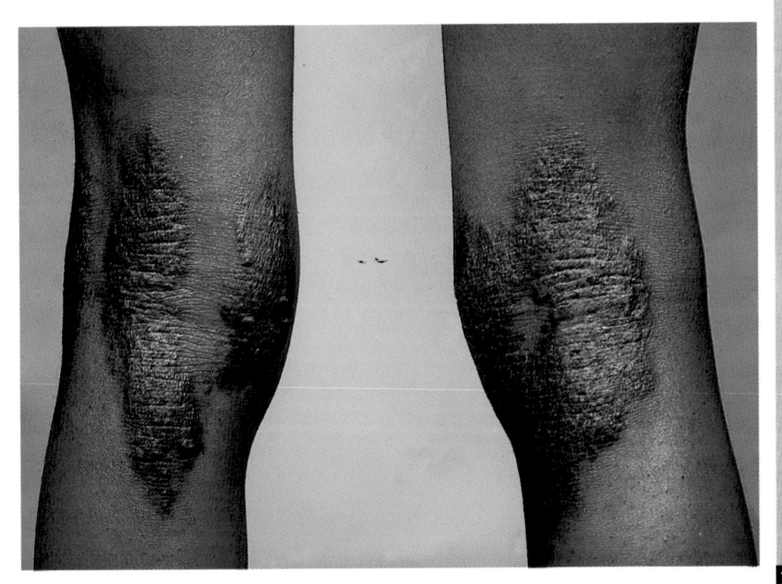

Fig. 44 Flexural lichenified eczema.

Reverse pattern The extensor surfaces of arms and legs are involved in some children. The pattern of eczema in these cases is frequently 'discoid' (Fig. 45). A 'papular' form of eczema is common in Afro-Caribbeans (Fig. 46).

Secondary infection This is common and eczema may be exacerbated through production of staphylococcal superantigen (Fig. 47).

Eczema herpeticum Herpes simplex (and in the past vaccinia) may disseminate widely in patients with atopic eczema (Fig. 48). Viral warts and molluscum contagiosum also occur more commonly in atopic persons.

Superficial, hypopigmented Patches of eczema affecting the face in children (Fig. 49, p. 33) (pityriasis alba) with or without involvement of trunk and limbs. It is not always associated with atopy. The condition is often more active in winter (low humidity) but more obvious in summer. It is poorly responsive to treatment but will improve with time. Emollients may help.

Keratosis pilaris (Fig. 50, p. 33) Is also sometimes associated with atopy. Follicular hyperkeratosis and erythema are seen particularly on upper outer arms and face.

Juvenile plantar dermatosis (forefoot eczema) Frictional and occlusive factors are important in this condition, as it seems to be a result of modern footwear. Atopic persons may be more susceptible. The feet have a characteristic glazed appearance with dryness and fissures (Fig. 51, p. 33).

'Nappy rash' Seborrhoeic napkin dermatitis may occasionally be the first manifestation of atopic eczema (see also pp. 10–13).

Irritant hand eczema Also more common in atopic individuals (Fig. 124, p. 79).

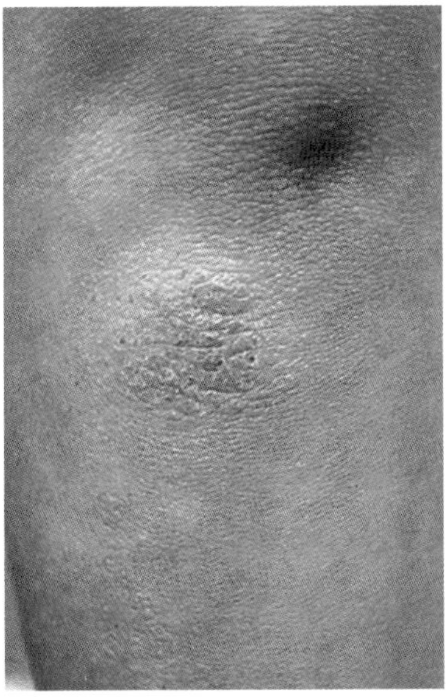

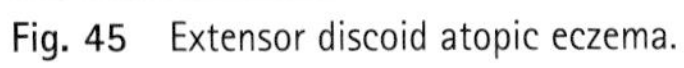

Fig. 45 Extensor discoid atopic eczema.

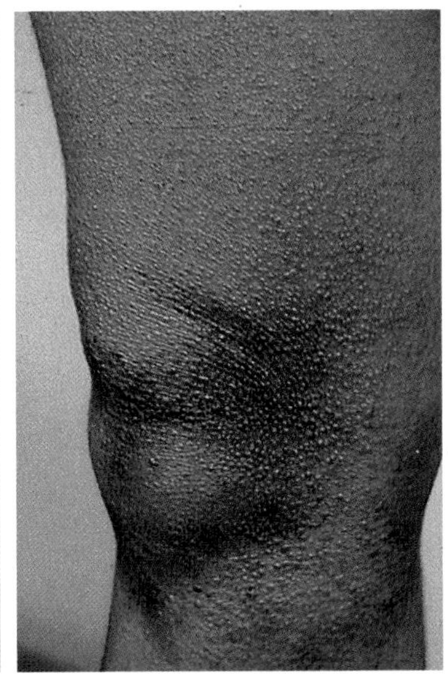

Fig. 46 Follicular/papular eczema.

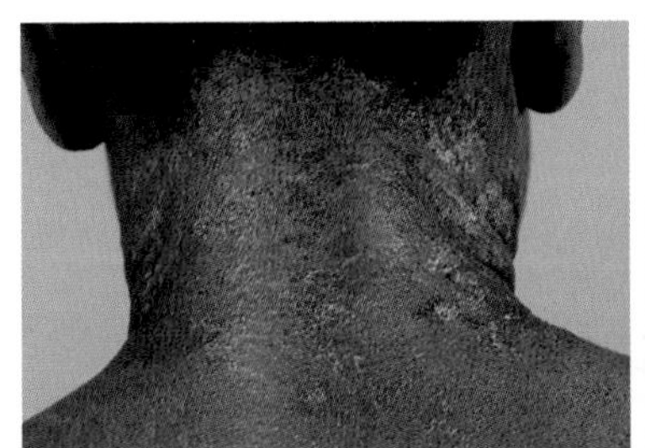

Fig. 47 Secondarily infected atopic eczema.

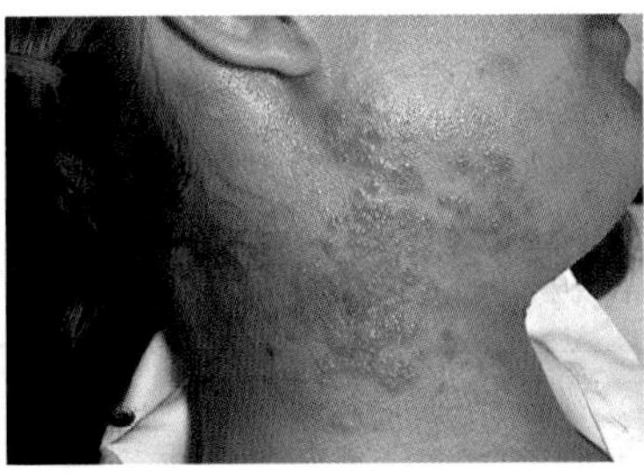

Fig. 48 Extensive herpes simplex in an atopic patient.

Management	
	Soap substitutes/water softeners/bath emollients Bath oils should be used; soaps and detergent must be avoided.

Emollients Oil in water creams, oily creams or ointments need to be used frequently to help hydrate the skin.

Tar preparations Coal tar paste or coal tar paste bandages are useful in chronic or lichenified eczema (applied on top of steroid).

Topical steroids Extremely effective. The potency of steroids used will depend on age, site, extent and activity of eczema. In general, hydrocortisone and clobetasone butyrate are preferred for children and facial or flexural skin, but short bursts of stronger steroids may be required to bring eczema under control.

Non-steroidal topical immunosuppressants Agents such as tacrolimus and pimecrolimus exhibit an efficacy equivalent to betamethasone and hydrocortisone and may therefore be useful for their steroid-sparing effects, especially at vulnerable sites.

Topical antibiotics May be required for infected eczema; these are often combined with a topical steroid. Systemic antibiotics are also often necessary.

Sedative antihistamines Help to reduce pruritus, especially at night.

Cotton clothing Preferable, as wool causes itching.

Wet wraps and compresses Helpful in the initial management of acute eczema.

Phototherapy Both PUVA and narrow-band UVB are helpful in chronic cases and for reducing dependence on steroids.

Systemic steroids Steroids or ciclosporin A only used in the most intractable and severe cases under expert supervision.

Chinese herbal treatment Also sometimes effective.

Systemic aciclovir Required for eczema herpeticum, which is a medical emergency.

Counselling Advice about the possible role of house dust mites, pets, dietary factors, etc., should be given to parents, and children should be given career advice so as to avoid irritant and wet work.

Habit reversal and cognitive therapy May help break the itch-scratch cycle.

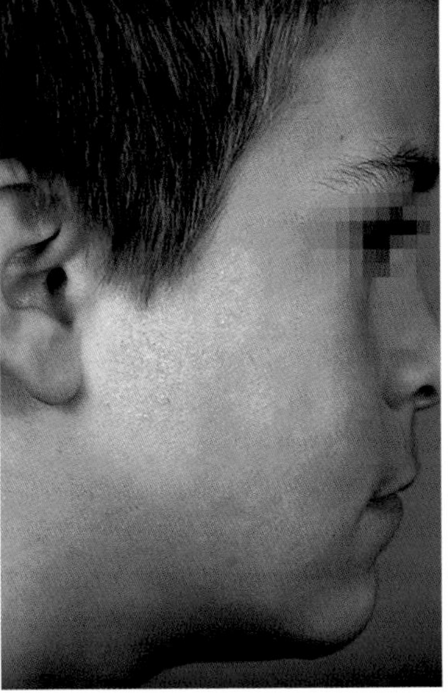

Fig. 49 Pityriasis alba (chronic superficial depigmenting dermatitis).

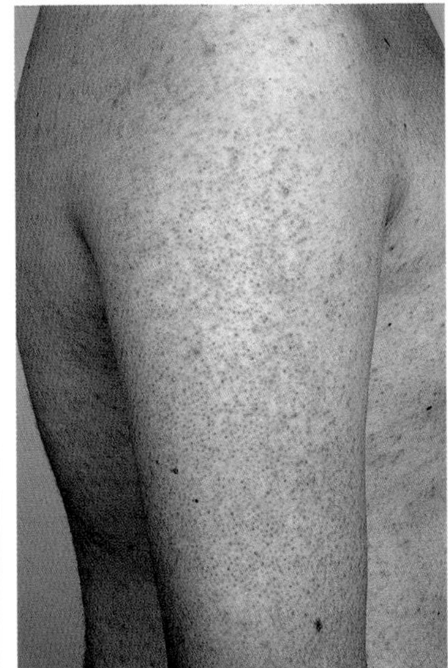

Fig. 50 Keratosis pilaris.

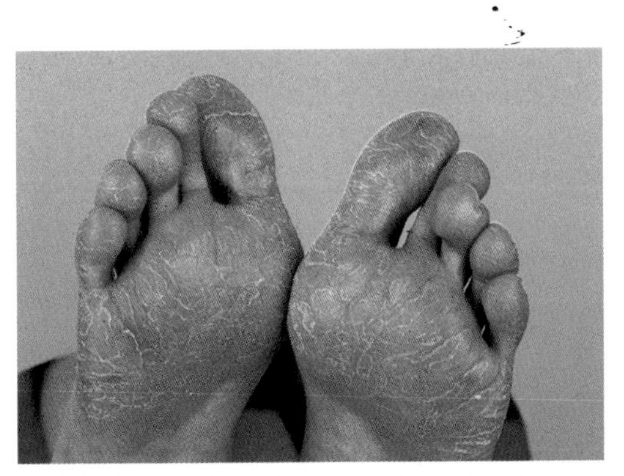

Fig. 51 Juvenile plantar dermatosis, the result of friction and occlusive footwear.

9 Urticaria and Henoch–Schönlein purpura

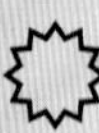

Acute urticaria (hives; nettle-rash)

Aetiology

Mast cell degranulation with histamine release due to drugs, foods, infections or infestations.

Clinical features

Increased incidence in atopic persons. Itchy wheals arise suddenly, within minutes, and last for some hours (Figs 52 & 53). There may be associated angioedema and eosinophilia.

Management

Treat any underlying infestation or infection. Antihistamines normally are helpful. Avoid colourings, all non-steroidal anti-inflammatory agents (NSAIDs), acetylsalicylic acid and any foods or drugs to which the patient is sensitive. Adrenaline (epinephrine) is needed if respiratory difficulties or anaphylaxis develops.

Henoch–Schönlein purpura (allergic vasculitis)

Aetiology

An immune complex hypersensitivity reaction to streptococcal infection.

Clinical features

Palpable (papular) purpura affects the lower legs, thighs and buttocks (Fig. 54); sometimes urticarial or necrotic. There may be arthralgia, abdominal pain, vomiting, and bloody diarrhoea. Renal damage may lead to proliferative glomerulonephritis with nephritic or nephrotic syndromes. Erythrocyte sedimentation rate (ESR) and anti-streptolysin O (ASO) titres may be raised.

The urine should be checked regularly for protein, casts and haematuria.

Management

Bed rest in the acute stage. Penicillin is administered for streptococcal infections; sometimes systemic steroids are used. Prognosis is generally good but depends on renal involvement.

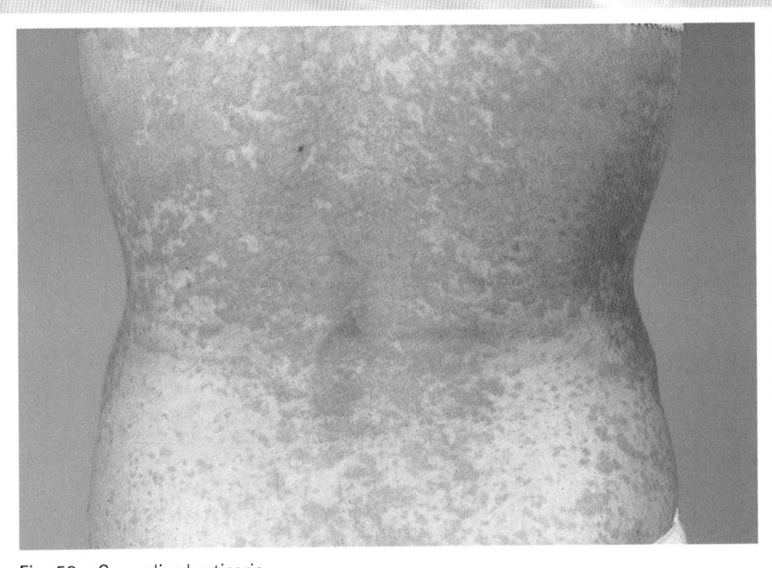

Fig. 52 Generalized urticaria.

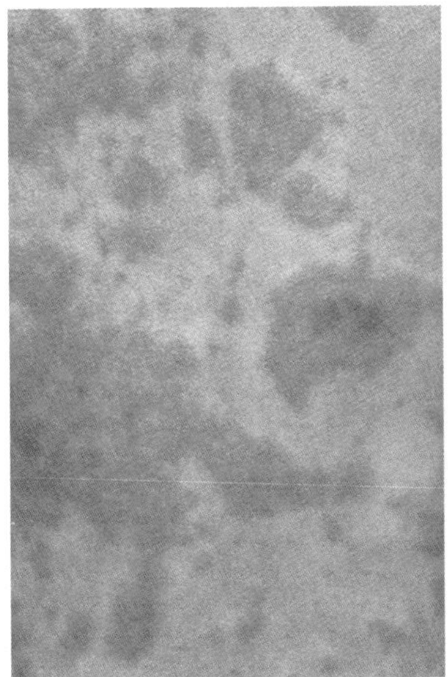

Fig. 53 Urticarial wheals

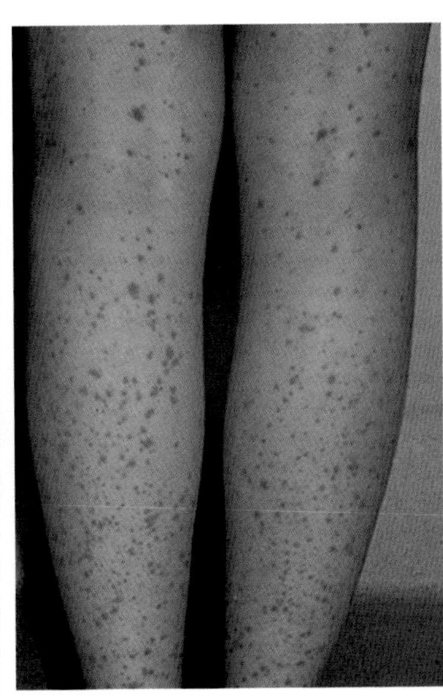

Fig. 54 Henoch–Schönlein type purpura.

10 Photosensitive eruptions

Polymorphic light eruption (PLE)

Clinical features

Relatively common; usually affects young women, although it may occur at any age; caused by intolerance to UVA; rash therefore develops in spite of window glass and UVB sunscreens. Itchy papules or papulovesicles, erythema and urticated plaques develop within hours, mainly at sites recently exposed to sun (Fig. 55). Starts in spring or early summer and declines thereafter. Tends to recur over many years. Sometimes associated with solar urticaria.

Management

Clothing and high protection broad-spectrum sunscreens or sunblocks. Topical steroids and oral antihistamines. Tolerance can be induced. PUVA or UVB therapy can be given prophylactically to thaose severely affected. Mepacrine, hydroxychloroquine or systemic steroids are sometimes required for severe cases.

Hutchinson's summer prurigo

Clinical features

Affects young children. There may be a family history. Itchy, erythematous, often excoriated papules on cheeks (Fig. 56), nose and dorsum of hands.

Management

Symptomatic. Sunscreens partially helpful.

Juvenile spring eruption

Clinical features

Uncommon condition seen in boys more frequently than girls. Erythema and pruritus of the ears is followed by grouped papules and vesicles. Cold may be a contributory factor.

Management

No treatment.

Skin disorders affected by sunlight

Aggravated Include polymorphic light eruption and other photodermatoses, lupus erythematosus (Fig. 57), dermatomyositis, porphyrias, rosacea, herpes simplex, erythema multiforme and benign lymphocytic infiltrations.

Helped Include psoriasis, acne vulgaris, pityriasis lichenoides, 'parapsoriasis' (both digitate dermatoses and mycosis fungoides).

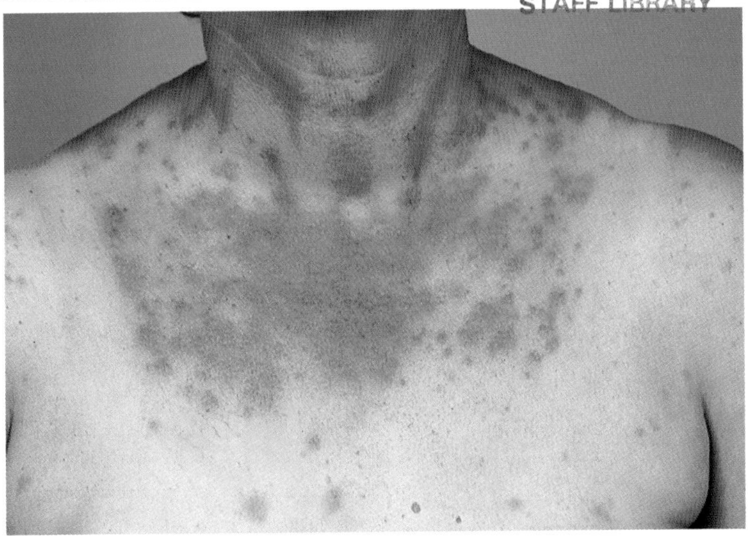

Fig. 55 Polymorphic light eruption.

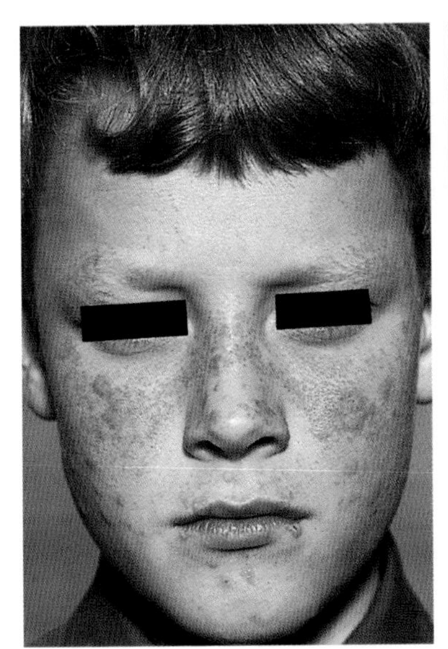

Fig. 56 Hutchinson's summer prurigo.

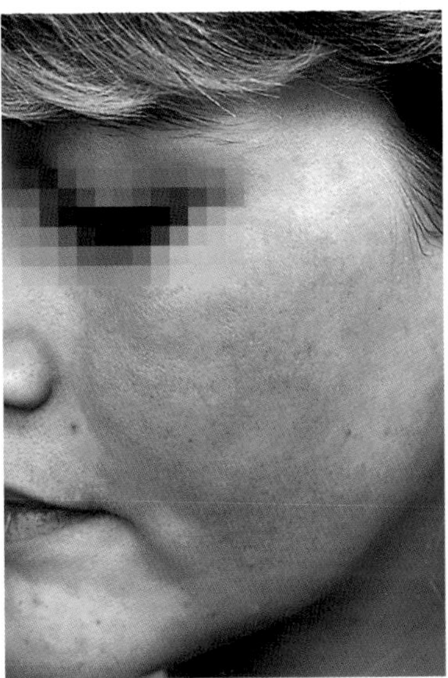

Fig. 57 Light aggravated, patchy, erythematous LE.

Photosensitive eczema

Aetiology

- Some eczemas (e.g. atopic and seborrhoeic dermatitis) may develop a secondary photosensitivity.
- Some topically applied chemicals (e.g. tar, creosote, plants) will cause phototoxic reactions.
- Certain systemic drugs (e.g. thiazides, phenothiazines, amiodarone and NSAIDs) may cause photosensitivity.
- Certain contact allergens, especially compositae, will cause chronic actinic dermatitis.

Clinical features

Mainly seen in the spring and summer. Drug-induced photosensitivity is normally due to long-wave UVL (UVA) (Fig. 58). Chronic actinic dermatitis is usually confined initially to short-wave UVL (UVB) exposed areas but in time may become chronic and extend to include UVA and visible light exposure, and it may be year-long and generalized.

Management

Elimination of drug and easily avoided environmental causes. In constitutional eczema or those sensitized to a ubiquitous allergen, symptomatic treatment with topical steroids and broad-spectrum sunscreens. In severe cases, systemic steroids, azathioprine or ciclosporin A.

Porphyria cutanea tarda (PCT)

Aetiology

An acquired or inherited form of porphyria associated with reduced hepatic uroporphyrinogen decarboxylase activity and increased porphyrins in plasma, urine and faeces. Often associated with alcohol abuse.

Clinical features

Vesicles, bullae, crusts and erosions (Fig. 59) develop on sun-exposed skin, often associated with milia, scarring, photosensitivity, increased skin fragility and hypertrichosis.

Management

Sun blocks; avoidance of alcohol, oestrogen and iron; regular venesection. In patients with unexplained photosensitivity, porphyrins and antinuclear factor (ANF) should always be checked.

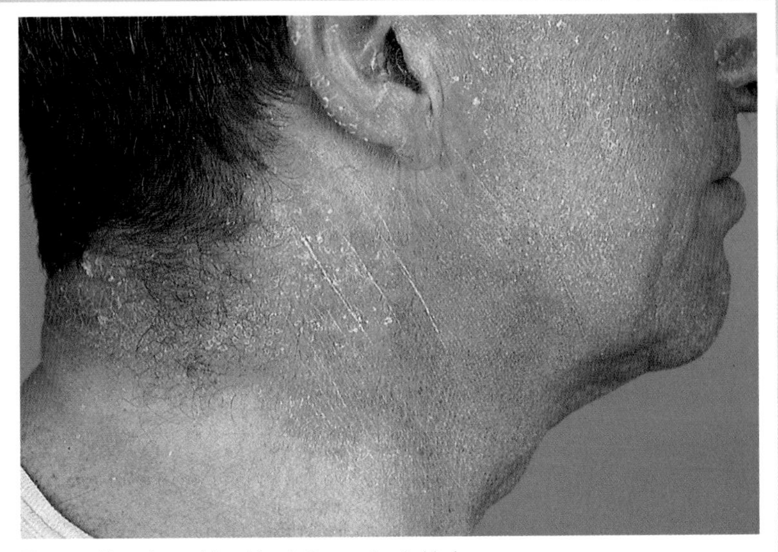

Fig. 58 Photodermatitis with relative sparing behind ear.

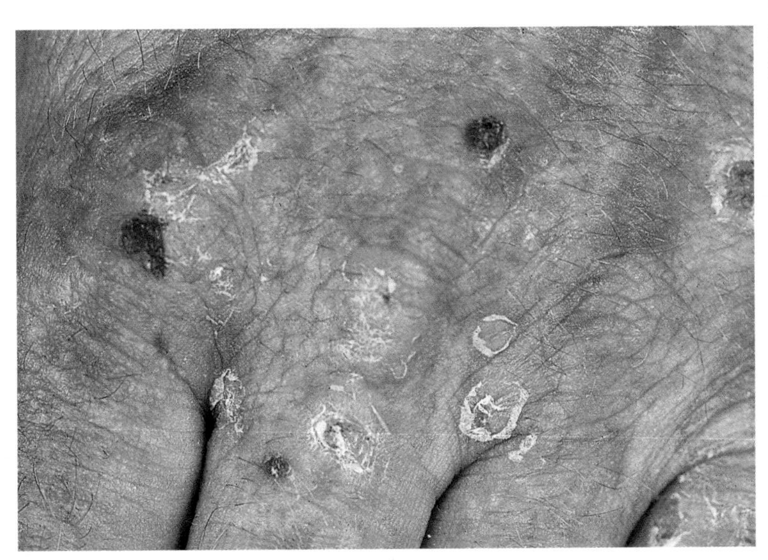

Fig. 59 Porphyria cutanea tarda.

11 Acne vulgaris

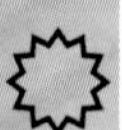

Acne is an inflammatory disorder of the pilosebaceous follicles, which occurs particularly at adolescence, when sebaceous glands become active.

Aetiology

Several factors are of importance:

- genetic
- androgenic (and, to some degree, progesterogenic) stimulation
- abnormal sebum production
- colonization of pilosebaceous unit with *Propionibacterium acnes*
- obstruction of the sebaceous duct
- inflammation.

Clinical features

The characteristic lesion is the *comedo* (plural, *comedones*) (Fig. 60), which appears as a dark follicular plug (blackhead) or a small cyst (closed comedo). Secondary inflammation causes papules and pustules, which may affect the face, chest, back and shoulders (Fig. 61). Premenstrual flares are common in women. Deeper *nodulocystic acne* (Fig. 62) occurs more commonly in men, as does *acne conglobata*, an uncommon, severe, recalcitrant form of acne with multiple 'paired' comedones and large (conglobate) cysts on the back, chest, neck and face. Scarring, including 'ice-pick' scarring (Fig. 63) may follow both acute superficial pustular acne and nodulocystic acne or acne conglobata (Figs 64 & 65, p. 43). Some individuals, especially Afro-Caribbeans, may have a tendency to develop hypertrophic or keloid scars (Fig. 66, p. 43).

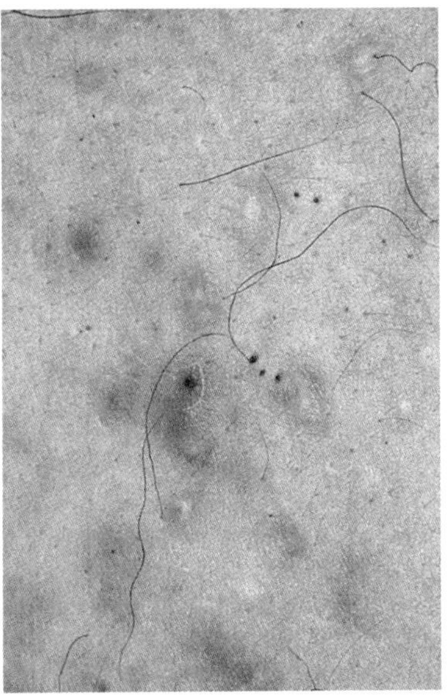

Fig. 60 Paired comedones as seen in acne conglobata.

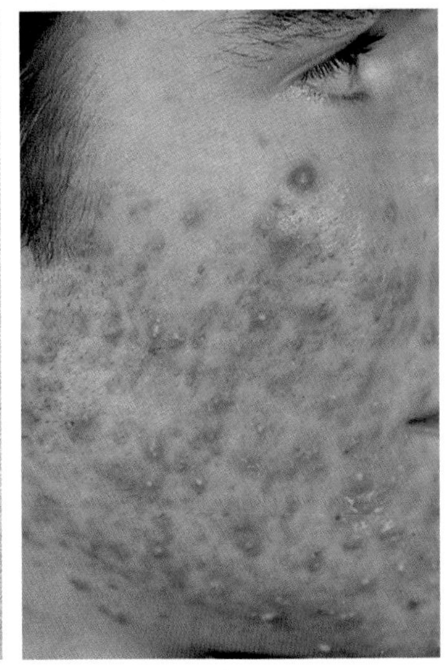

Fig. 61 Superficial inflammatory acne.

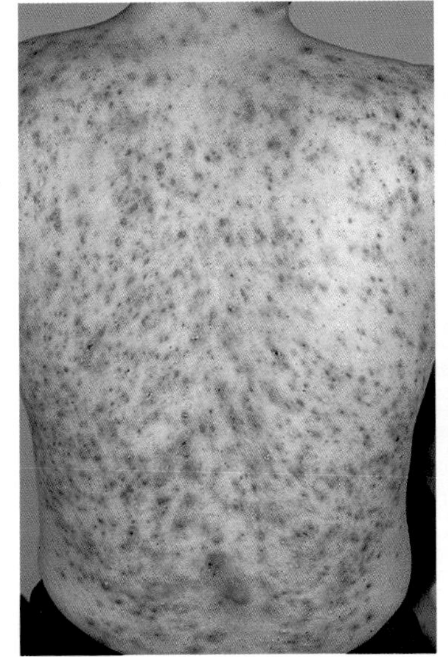

Fig. 62 Severe, extensive acne (acne conglobata).

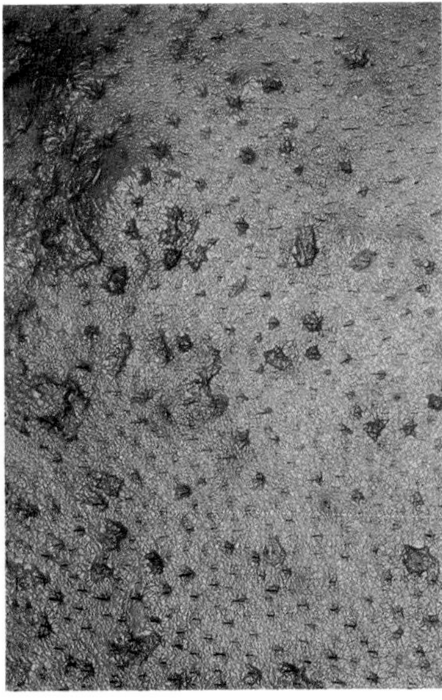

Fig. 63 'Ice-pick' scarring.

Management

Topical therapy

Keratolytics Beneficial for superficial acne.

Benzoyl peroxide Both antibacterial and drying or peeling action.

Tretinoin/isotretinoin/adapalene Useful for comedonal acne. Intermittent use is recommended initially.

Topical antibiotics Agents such as erythromycin, clindamycin and tetracycline in a propylene glycol and spirit base are of benefit in superficial inflammatory acne.

Ultraviolet light and natural sunlight Often beneficial; produce erythema and slight peeling.

Systemic therapy

Oral antibiotics Oxytetracycline or erythromycin, 500 mg b.d., produces improvement in about 70% of patients. For tetracycline, it is important that therapy be taken with water and away from food. For maintenance therapy, antibiotics may be given at lower dose. They will need to be continued for some months or years. Once-daily tetracyclines, such as lymecycline, are now available. Minocycline is useful when there is tetracycline resistance. (NB: avoid tetracyclines during pregnancy and breast-feeding and until second dentition is complete.)

Oral contraceptives Some contraceptive pills, such as those containing cyproterone acetate plus ethinylestradiol or drospirenone or desogestrel plus ethylstilbestrol, may be helpful in patients with acne.

Oral retinoids (13-*cis*-retinoic acid) Can produce a dramatic improvement in acne. Teratogenic side-effects limit its use in women, and the treatment is at present only available from dermatologists for severe or resistant acne in men or women on secure contraception.

Steroids Topical steroids are contraindicated; intralesional steroids are used for acne keloid and sometimes half-strength for inflammatory nodulocystic lesions. Short courses of oral steroids are only rarely used for acute inflammatory acne or acne fulminans.

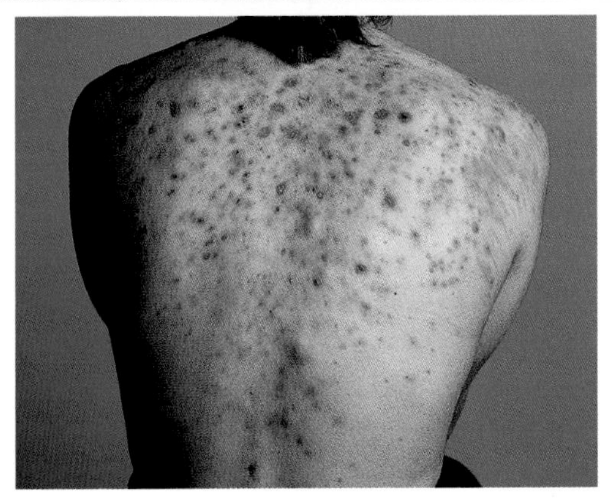

Fig. 64 Extensive acne and scarring.

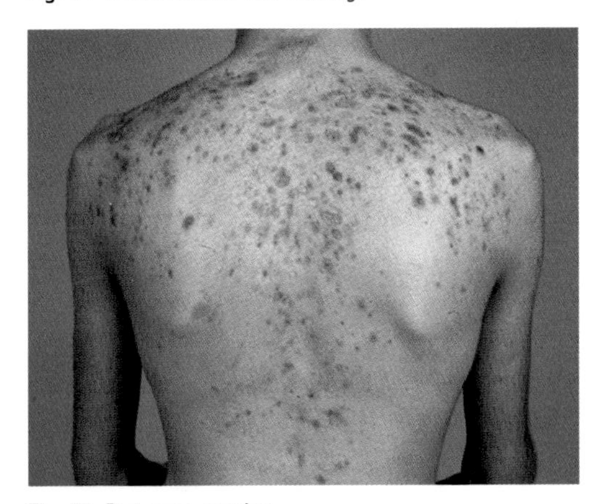

Fig. 65 Post-acne scarring.

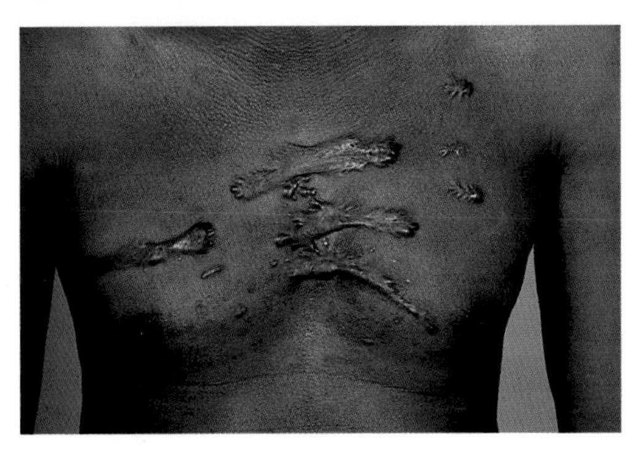

Fig. 66 Keloid scars.

12 Rosacea

Aetiology

Unknown. Increased lability and reactivity of the facial vasculature.

Clinical features

Initially, transient flushing but later a persistent and diffuse facial erythema with inflamed papules and pustules (acne rosacea) (Fig. 67) and telangiectasia. Chiefly involves glabella, cheeks, nose and chin. Lymphoedema, conjunctival suffusion, conjunctivitis, blepharitis and (rarely) keratitis are seen. It may be exacerbated by sun, heat, alcohol and hot or spicy foods. It is more common in women, especially those with fair skin or Celtic inheritance.

Rhinophyma (Fig. 68) is a variant seen mainly in men, in which there is enlargement of the nose due to hypertrophy of sebaceous glands.

Management

Avoid precipitating factors. Oral tetracyclines (papules and pustules). Topical 1% metronidazole cream for mild cases. Low dose antibiotics needed for months or years. Topical steroids are contraindicated. Rhinophyma usually requires plastic surgery.

Perioral dermatitis

Aetiology

Unknown. It may develop from paraoral acne or paranasal seborrhoeic dermatitis. Prior use of a potent topical steroid is usually a factor.

Clinical features

Papulopustular eruption on a scaly, erythematous background around the mouth, nose and nasolabial folds. It is more frequent in women (Fig. 69).

Management

Systemic oxytetracycline or erythromycin (a reducing 4–6 week course), with 1% hydrocortisone cream initially to reduce 'rebound' when potent steroids are withdrawn (if necessary) or topical 1% metronidazole cream or clindamycin aqueous lotion in those unable to tolerate systemic antibiotics. (NB: avoid tetracycline and metronidazole in woman who are pregnant or breast-feeding.)

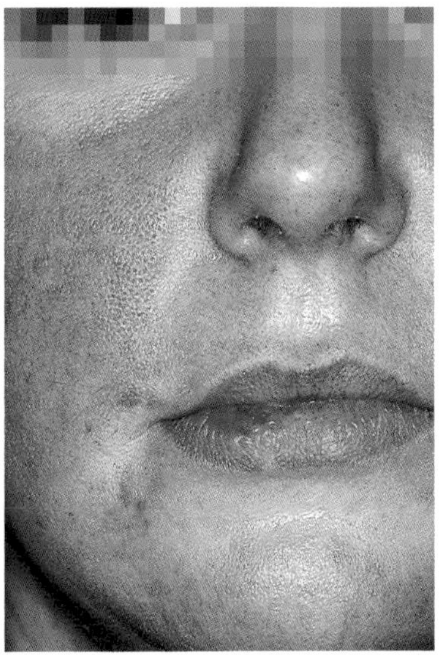

Fig. 67 Acne rosacea.

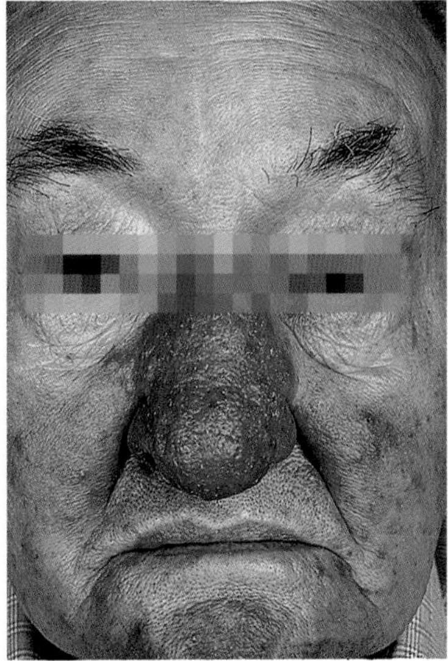

Fig. 68 Rhinophyma.

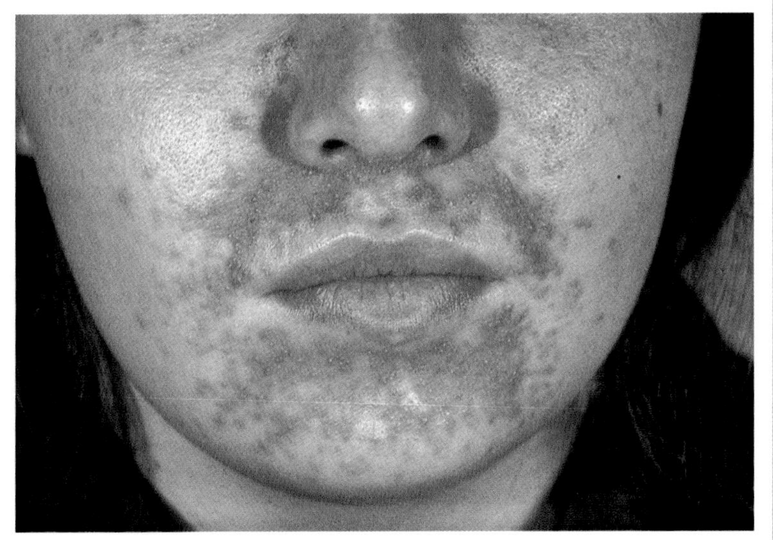

Fig. 69 Perioral dermatitis.

13 Psoriasis

Aetiology

Psoriasis affects approximately 2% of the population. Genetic factors are important: 40% of patients have a positive family history. There is a rapid epidermal transit time with increased epidermal cell production.

Clinical features

Plaque psoriasis Characterized by well-demarcated, erythematous areas covered with thick, silvery scales (Fig. 70). Pinpoint capillary bleeding occurs when scales are removed. Symmetrical plaques commonly affect extensor surfaces, especially the elbows and knees (Fig. 71). The condition frequently affects the scalp and sacrum (Fig. 72), but patches may occur anywhere on the body and at sites of trauma (Köbner phenomenon) (Fig. 73).

Guttate (and exanthematic) psoriasis (Figs 74–76, p. 49) Common in the young and often precipitated by a streptococcal sore throat. Multiple 'rain-drop' lesions occur suddenly on trunk and limbs. The condition may resolve spontaneously, or individual spots may enlarge and turn into plaque psoriasis.

Pustular psoriasis Rare generalized form which can be fatal. Patients are often erythrodermic with sheets of sterile pustules (Fig. 77, p. 49) and associated fever, malaise and leukocytosis. Localized forms also exist.

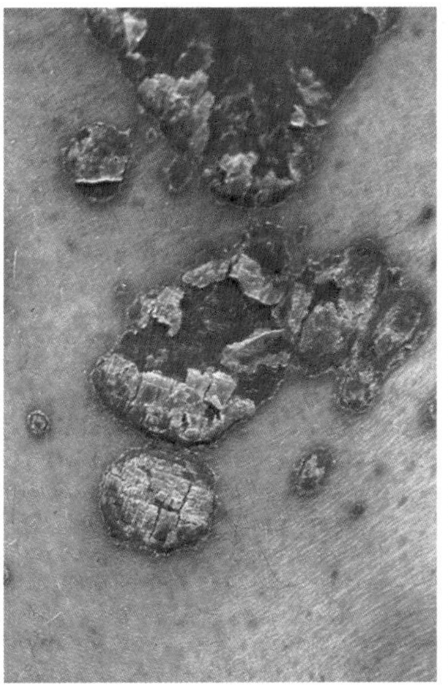

Fig. 70 Typical psoriatic plaques with thick silvery scales.

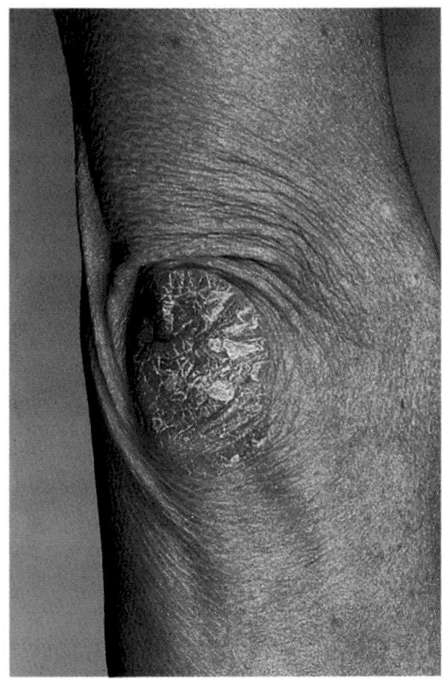

Fig. 71 Typical psoriasis on elbow.

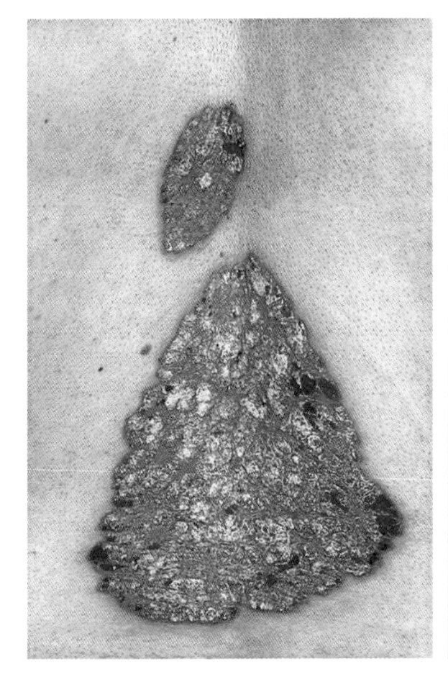

Fig. 72 Psoriatic plaque.

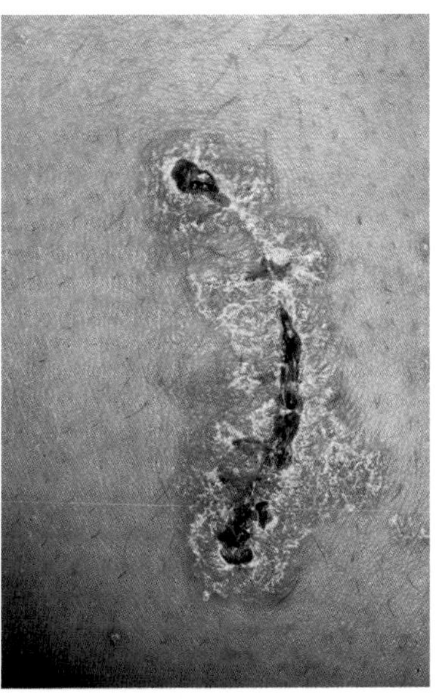

Fig. 73 Psoriasis showing Köbner phenomenon.

Flexural psoriasis The affected psoriatic skin loses its characteristic silvery scale, but the well-demarcated erythematous areas (Fig. 78, p. 51) remain and may mimic intertrigo, candidiasis and tinea.

Erythrodermic psoriasis When psoriasis involves the whole body, the resulting erythroderma may be difficult to differentiate from other types of erythrodermic exfoliative dermatoses (Fig. 79, p. 51). Such patients lose their ability to control body temperature and fluid balance and are at risk for both infection and cardiac and renal failure.

Persistent palmoplantar pustulosis This is often regarded as a localized form of psoriasis of the hands and feet, but it frequently occurs without evidence of psoriasis elsewhere. Common in smokers. Localized patches of erythema and scaling occur on the palms and soles (Fig. 80, p. 51) with scattered, sterile, yellow-brown pustules. The condition is very resistant to treatment.

Scalp psoriasis Multiple discrete plaques or involvement of the entire scalp with or without ears and scalp margins. Plaques are frequently thick, particularly at the occiput, but alopecia is uncommon.

Nail psoriasis The nails are commonly affected by several abnormalities in psoriasis, including pitting, onycholysis, subungual hyperkeratosis, wax spots (p. 140).

Psoriatic arthropathy Commonly affects the terminal interphalangeal joints and sacroiliac joints, but both large and small joints may be involved. A severe, destructive form of arthritis known as 'arthritis mutilans' is occasionally seen.

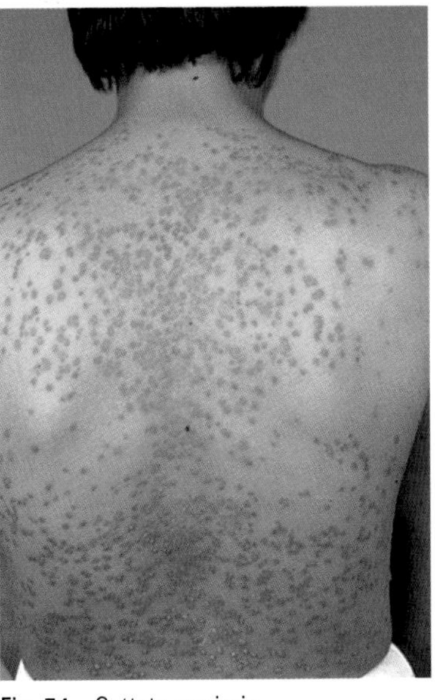

Fig. 74 Guttate psoriasis.

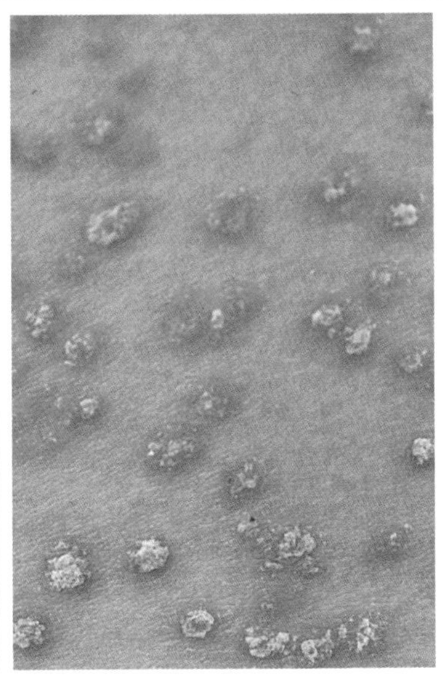

Fig. 75 Guttate psoriasis: raindrop lesions.

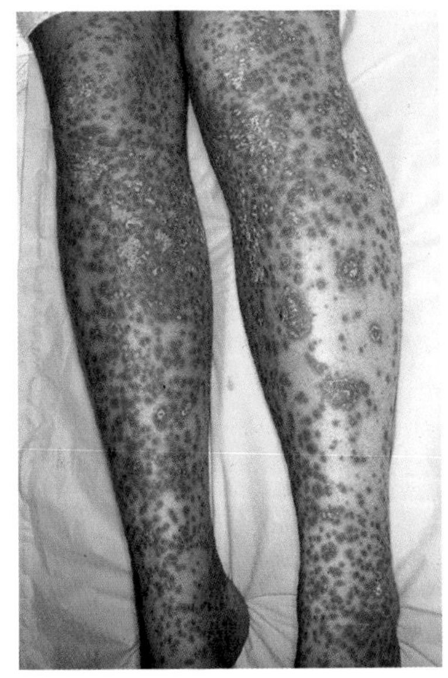

Fig. 76 Exanthematic psoriasis.

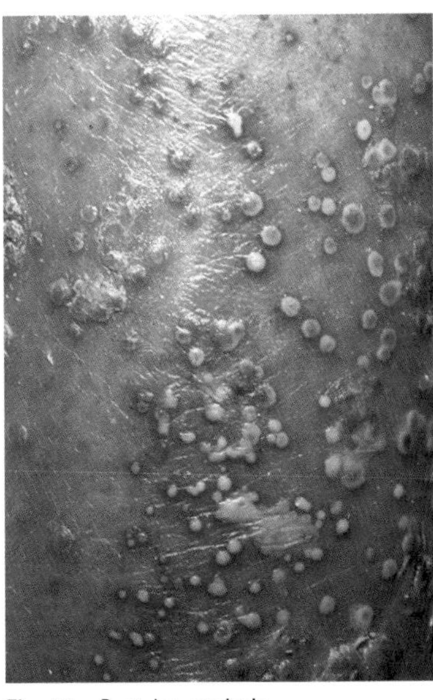

Fig. 77 Pustular psoriasis.

Management

Topical steroids Effective, but continued use may lead to lessening of effect and some destabilization of ordinary plaque psoriasis. These are better employed (in a descending sequence of potency) in combination with tar, topical vitamin D (calcipotriol) or topical retinoids (tazarotene). This combines the rapid initial benefits and cosmetic acceptability of topical steroids (by day) with the slower but more long-lasting effects of other preparations (at night). Weaker steroid preparations remain very useful for intertriginous areas.

Tar Can be used either alone or combined with salicylic acid. Cleaner forms are now available.

Ultraviolet light E_0–E_1 doses of UVB alone or combined with tar or tar baths or newer treatments using narrow-band UVB. Psoralen with UVA (PUVA) is successful at clearing extensive refractory psoriasis.

Dithranol Useful for plaque psoriasis in inpatients. It is diluted in Lassar's paste, initially at 0.1% and then at increased strength. Cleaner forms are now available for outpatient use applied for just half-an-hour and then washed off. Treatment may be combined with tar baths and UVB.

Vitamin D_3 (calcipotriol/calcitriol/tacalcitol) Topical treatments for psoriasis, with an efficacy equivalent to that of topical steroids, but with slower response. Only 70% effective in 70% of cases on its own, but can be combined with both topical phototherapy and topical steroids.

Systemic therapy Cytotoxic drugs (e.g. methotrexate, ciclosporin or etretinate, etc.) are treatments normally only initiated by dermatologists.

Scalp psoriasis regimens Keratolytics, tar shampoos, topical steroids as lotions or gels. Vitamin D_3 also available as scalp preparation.

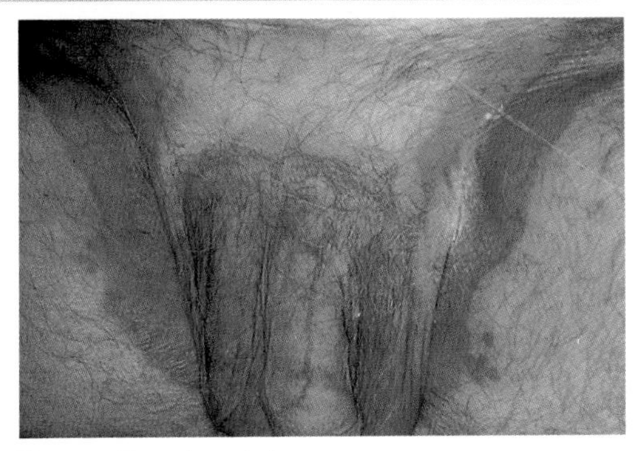

Fig. 78 Flexural psoriasis.

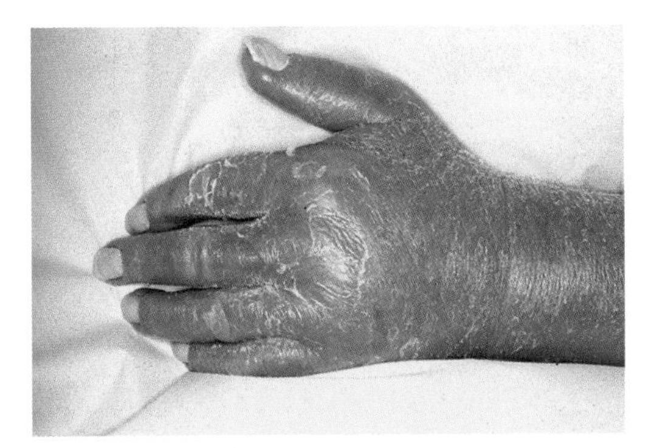

Fig. 79 Exfoliative/erythrodermic psoriasis.

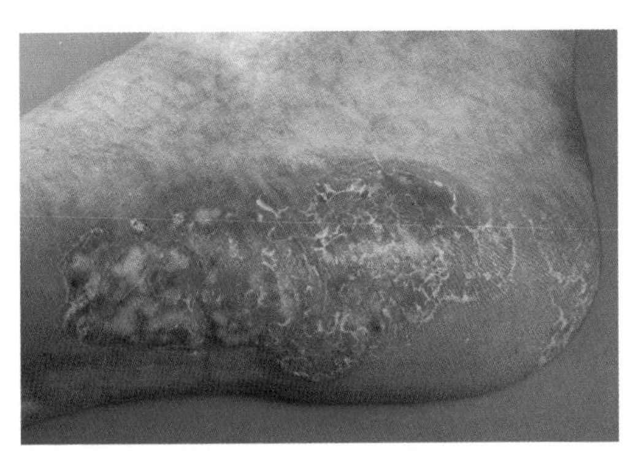

Fig. 80 Persistent palmoplantar pustulosis.

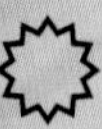

14 Pityriasis

Pityriasis rosea

Aetiology

The cause is unknown; an infective agent has been suggested but not isolated.

Clinical features

Common, self-limiting eruption which predominantly affects young adults. Characteristically, the initial lesion is a solitary oval, erythematous, scaly 'herald patch', often on the trunk (Fig. 81) and often mistaken for a fungal infection. Similar but smaller lesions appear after an interval of 1 or 2 weeks over the trunk, neck and upper arms in a symmetrical and generalized distribution. Individual lesions lie parallel to the ribs, creating a 'Christmas tree' pattern (Fig. 82). Pruritus is minimal, but occasionally there may be malaise and lymphadenopathy. The eruption usually fades within 4–6 weeks.

Management

Usually no treatment is required. Mild topical steroids may hasten resolution and help the more 'eczematous' cases.

Pityriasis lichenoides

Aetiology

Unknown.

Clinical features

Two forms exist: acute and chronic.

Acute Adolescents are usually affected. Small, red papules occur on the trunk and limbs. The lesions become vesicular and necrotic and ulcerate to leave pitted scars. Fever and systemic upset may occur. Mucous membranes may be involved. The eruption is often mistaken for chickenpox (Fig. 83).

Chronic Small, reddish or orange-brown papules. Some may be purpuric, others develop a characteristic 'mica' scale. Lesions resolve slowly, leaving either a brown hyperpigmented or hypopigmented mark (Fig. 84). There is no systemic upset. The condition may persist for months or years.

Management

None may be necessary. Ultraviolet light (UVB), PUVA and sunshine are all useful in the chronic form. There are reports that erythromycin may be effective.

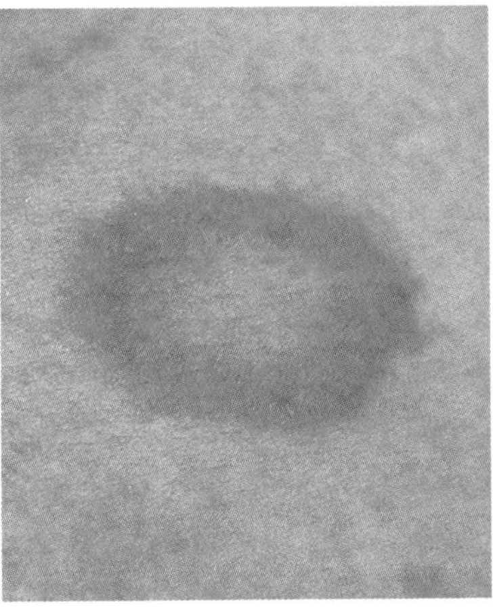

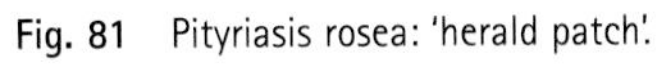

Fig. 81 Pityriasis rosea: 'herald patch'.

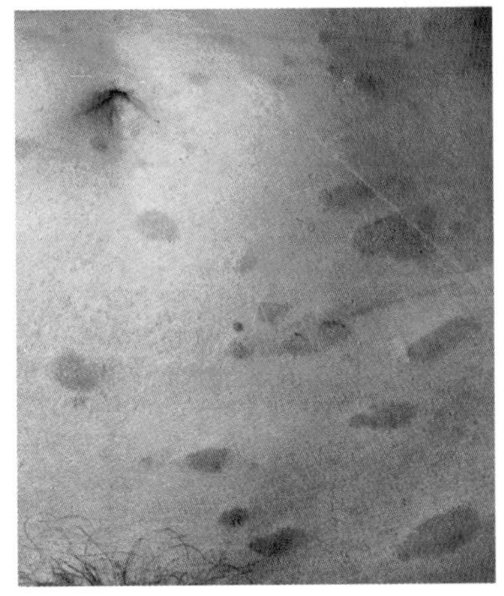

Fig. 82 Typical distribution of lesions in pityriasis rosea.

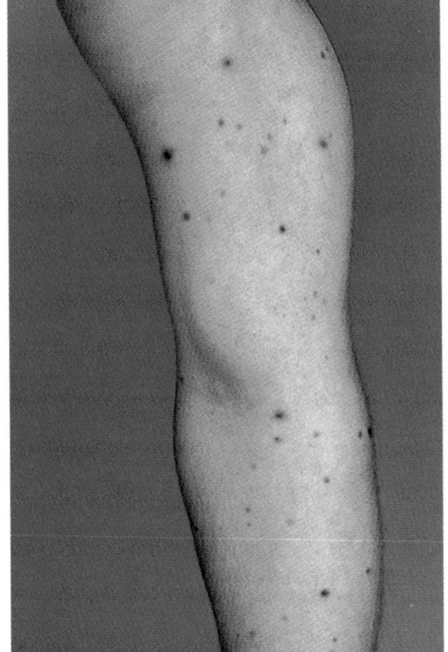

Fig. 83 Pityriasis lichenoides acuta.

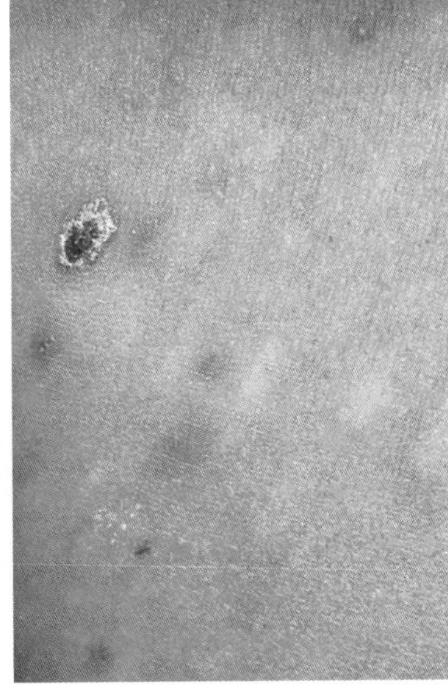

Fig. 84 Pityriasis lichenoides chronica with post-inflammatory hypopigmentation.

Sarcoidosis

Aetiology	Unknown. A multisystem, granulomatous disease.
Clinical features	*Erythema nodosum* See page 68. *Lupus pernio* (Fig. 85) Indurated, soft, blue-red plaques affect nose, ears, fingers, cheeks. *Papulonodular* Firm, blue-red papules, nodules or plaques affect the face, trunk and extensor surfaces of limbs (Fig. 86). Annular lesions also occur. *Scar sarcoid* Existing scars may become infiltrated.
Management	Oral steroids if systemic symptoms warrant.

Annular erythema

Aetiology	Often idiopathic. Drugs, infections and carcinoma have been implicated. Variants include erythema chronicum migrans (tick bite), erythema gyratum repens (underlying carcinoma) and erythema marginatum (active rheumatic fever). Rule out subacute lupus erythematosus (LE).
Clinical features	Small, pink papules enlarge slowly to form ring or polycyclic patterns with central clearing (Fig. 87). They may be solitary or multiple, lasting weeks or months.
Management	None; tetracyclines if Lyme disease is suspected.

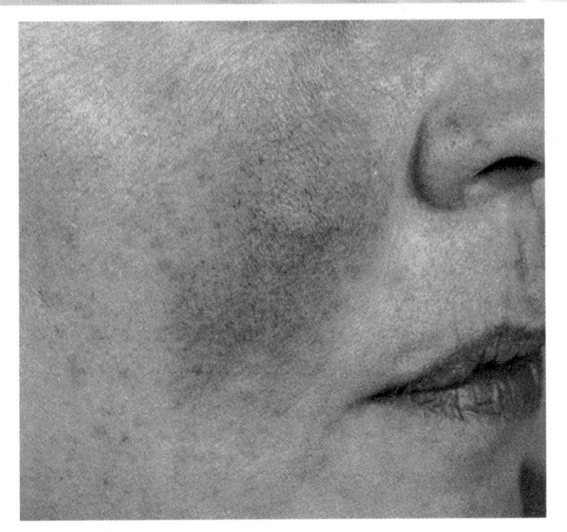

Fig. 85 Lupus pernio.

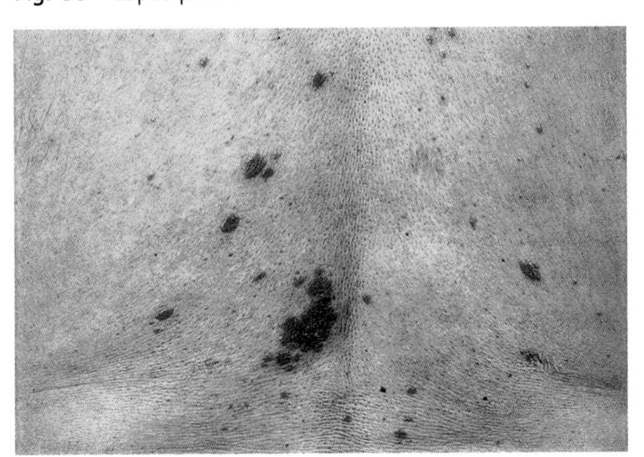

Fig. 86 Cutaneous sarcoid.

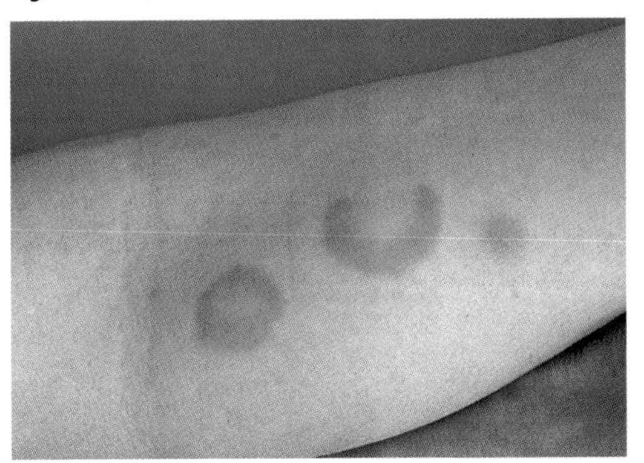

Fig. 87 Annular erythema.

Granuloma annulare

Aetiology

Unknown. May rarely be associated with diabetes mellitus.

Clinical features

Commonly affects children. Solitary or multiple firm, smooth, skin-coloured or violaceous papules appear on the dorsum of hands or feet (Fig. 88), fingers, ankles, elbows and elsewhere. Typically they progress into annular lesions. Most resolve spontaneously within 1–2 years. More diffuse and persistent form seen in adults (Fig. 89).

Management

None. Potent steroids with occlusion; intralesional corticosteroids rarely.

Necrobiosis lipoidica

Aetiology

Unknown. Some cases are associated with diabetes.

Clinical features

A reddish-brown, slowly enlarging plaque with shiny, yellow, atrophic centre (Fig. 90), classically involving the front of the shins. Lesions show telangiectasia and some eventually ulcerate. Differential diagnosis: granuloma annulare, basal cell carcinoma.

Management

Test for diabetes. Potent topical steroids (with or without occlusion). Intralesional steroids are of some value.

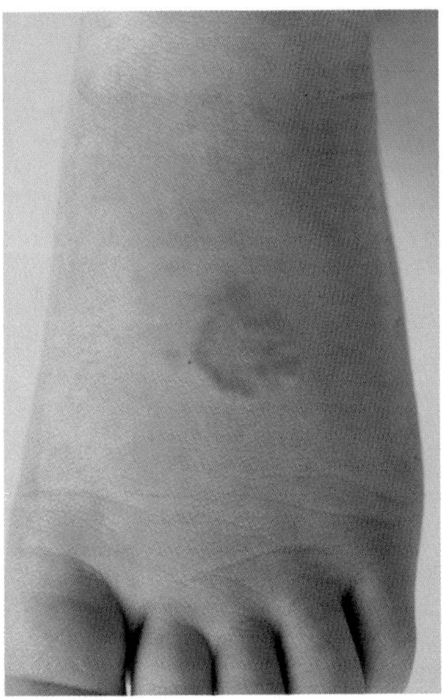

Fig. 88 Granuloma annulare, classical childhood type.

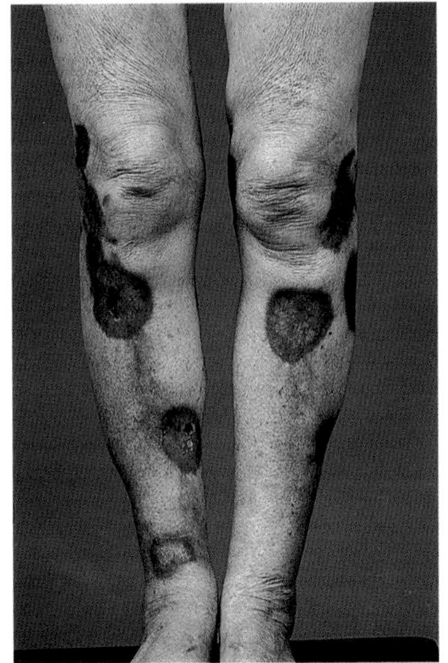

Fig. 90 Necrobiosis lipoidica.

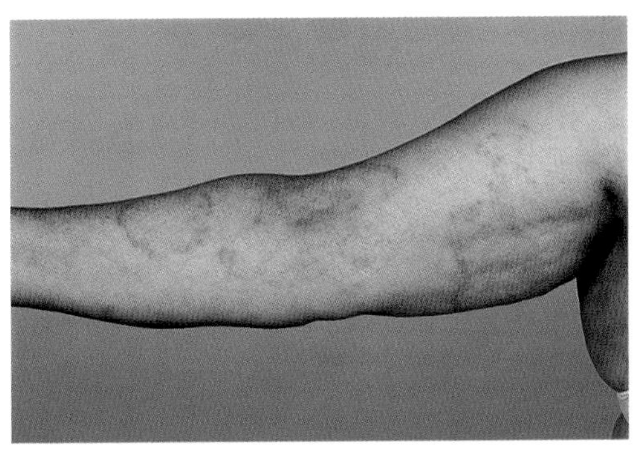

Fig. 89 Diffuse adult type granuloma annulare.

Keloids/hypertrophic scars

Aetiology

Excess proliferation of dermal collagen. Risk is increased with tension, infection or foreign material. There is occasionally a family history. Hypertrophic scars commoner in Afro-Caribbean persons.

Clinical features

Firm, raised, smooth, pink (or brown) plaques or nodules develop 4–6 weeks after skin trauma, particularly on the ear lobe after ear-piercing (Fig. 91), and on the upper back, shoulders, neck and presternal areas. Keloids tend to spread beyond the original injury (Fig. 66, p. 43).

Management

Intralesional steroids or potent topical steroids under occlusion may help. Silastic dressings, silicone gels and compression garments may help in the early phase of development.

Dermatofibroma

A localized fibrotic tissue response to insect bites (Fig. 92).

Xanthomatosis (hyperlipidaemias)

Aetiology

Localized cutaneous deposits of lipid. The condition may be primary or secondary to diabetes, myxoedema, pancreatitis and nephrotic syndrome.

Clinical features

Xanthelasma Symmetrical, firm, flat, yellow plaques affecting the upper and lower eyelids (Fig. 93). There is usually no lipid abnormality; some affected persons have type II hyperlipidaemia with raised cholesterol levels and a positive family history.

Xanthomata Firm, yellowish nodules over the knees, elbows (Fig. 94), heels and buttocks. Tendon xanthomas occur in types II and III hyperlipidaemia.

Eruptive xanthomata Small, yellow or red-brown papules occurring on the buttocks and extensor surfaces of the limbs; characteristic in type I and V hyperlipidaemias but also common in type IV hyperlipidaemia.

Management

Treat underlying hyperlipidaemia.

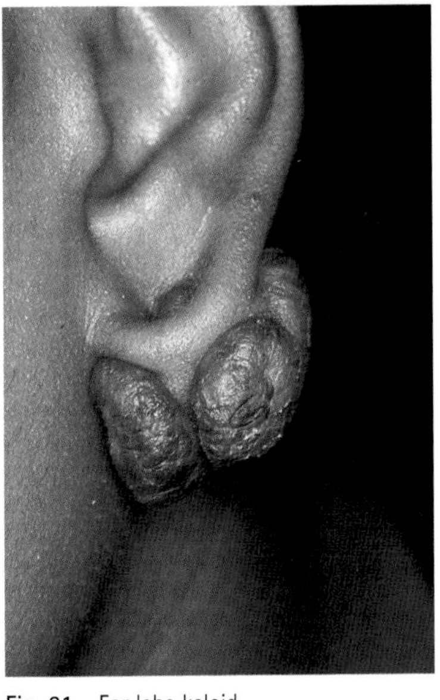
Fig. 91 Ear lobe keloid.

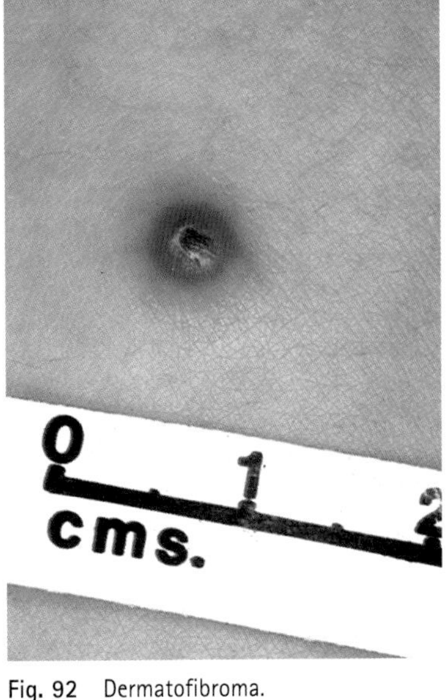

Fig. 92 Dermatofibroma.

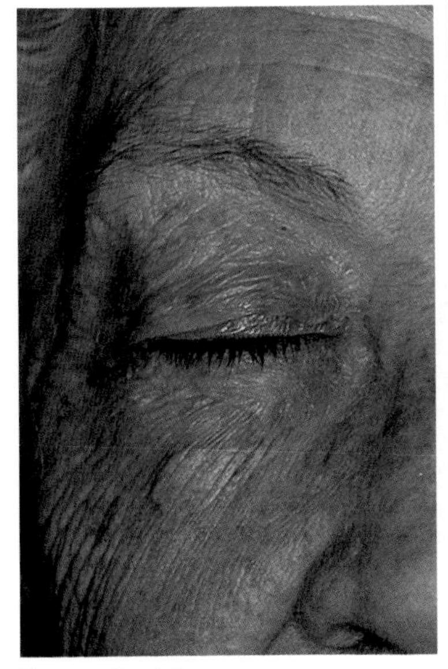
Fig. 93 Xanthelasma.

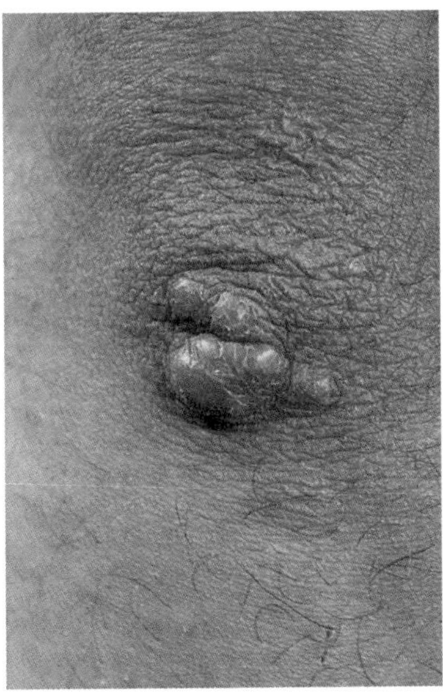
Fig. 94 Tuberous xanthoma.

16 Urticaria and angioedema

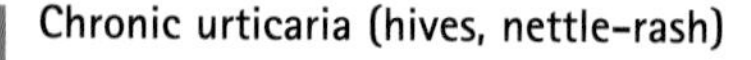

Chronic urticaria (hives, nettle-rash)

Aetiology

An increase in vascular permeability or reactivity. Both immune and non-immune (pharmacological) mechanisms may play a part. Histamine is only one of several mediators. Most cases are autoimmune or idiopathic. Precipitating factors include

- drugs (e.g. aspirin, NSAIDs)
- food additives (e.g. tartrazine [E102])
- infections
- stress
- disorders of the immune system (e.g. systemic lupus erythematosus [SLE], complement deficiency)
- infections (e.g. thrush)
- infestations (e.g. parasites and intestinal worms)

In many cases no obvious cause is found.

Clinical features

Transient raised wheals varying from a few millimetres to several centimetres in size (Figs 95 & 96). Limbs and trunk are particularly affected, but lesions may occur anywhere. Wheals are extremely itchy, last from 4–24 h and fade completely. Pressure sites are commonly affected, and most patients are also dermographic. There may be associated angioedema. Rarely, chronic urticaria may overlap with urticarial vasculitis (Fig. 97).

Management

Avoid acetylsalicylic acid and any other drugs that may have been implicated. Treat any underlying bacterial, fungal or parasitic infection. Low fat, dye-free and preservative-free diets may help. Antihistamines give relief; severely affected patients may require systemic steroids.

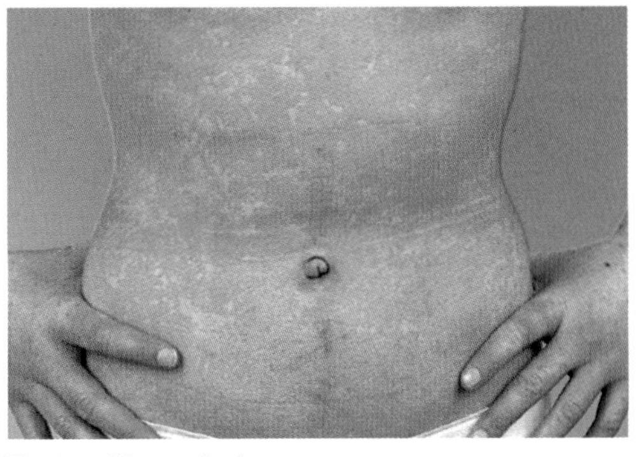

Fig. 95 Giant urticaria.

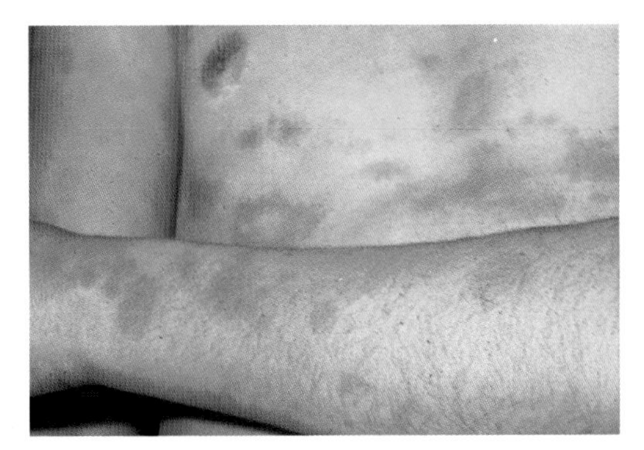

Fig. 96 Urticarial wheals.

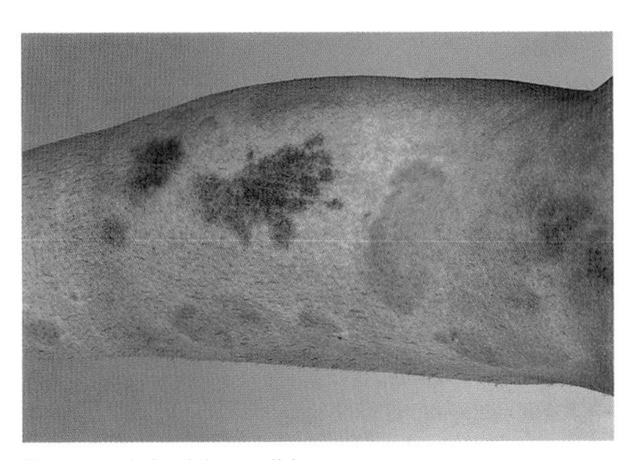

Fig. 97 Urticarial vasculitis.

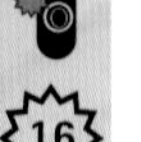

Angioedema

Aetiology

Hereditary angioedema is an autosomal dominant condition due to C1 esterase inhibitor deficiency in the complement cascade. Angioedema may also occur as part of the symptom complex in both acute and chronic urticaria. Nuts and fish or shellfish are the most common dietary allergic causes.

Clinical features

Angioedema produces swelling of the lips (Figs 98 & 99), periorbital area (Fig. 100), neck and joints. The larynx may be affected, and such involvement can be fatal. Gut involvement may produce abdominal pains. Urticaria is not normally a feature of true hereditary angioedema but angioedema may occur in cases of ordinary urticaria.

Management

Anyone who suffers recurrent attacks of angioedema or in whom there is a family history of angioedema should be positively screened for C1 esterase inhibitor deficiency. Measurement of C4 is a good screening test. Specific drugs such as stanozolol, tranexamic acid and danazol are the only effective prophylactic agents for hereditary angioedema. Acute episodes require injection of C1 esterase inhibitor or infusion of fresh frozen plasma. Angioedema associated with ordinary urticaria may be treated with antihistamines (with or without steroids). Severe attacks should be treated as for anaphylaxis, with 0.5 ml 1:1000 adrenaline (epinephrine) by intramuscular injection.

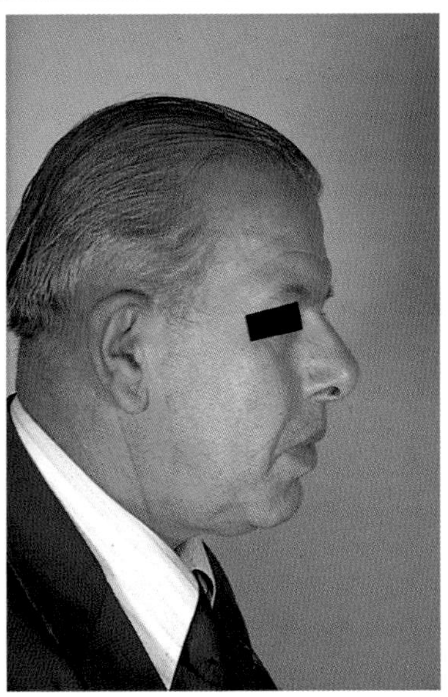

Fig. 98 Acetylsalicylic acid-induced angioedema (before).

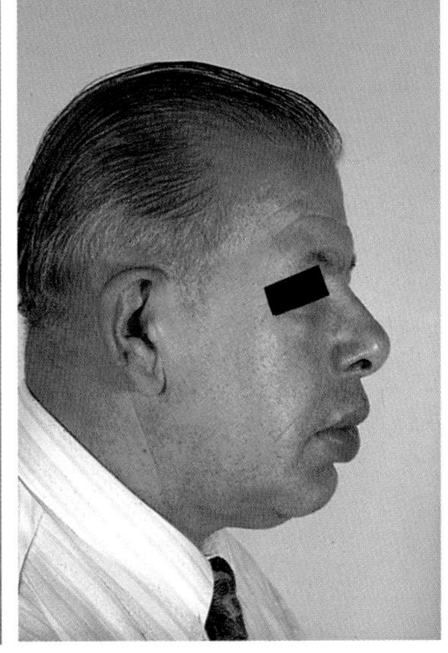

Fig. 99 Acetylsalicylic acid-induced angioedema (after).

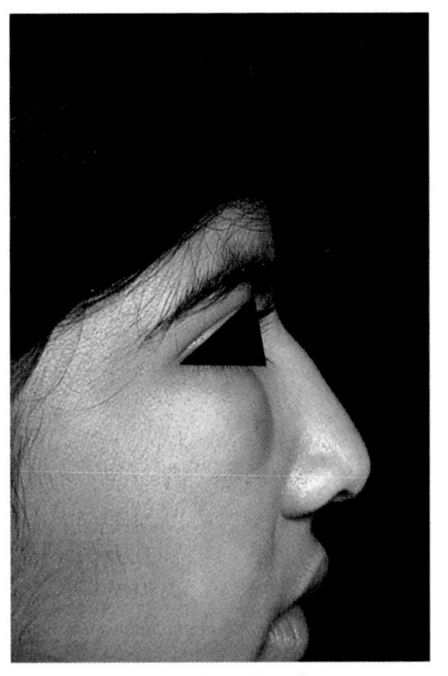

Fig. 100 Periorbital swelling (recurrent angioedema).

17 Physical urticarias

Dermographism

Clinical features

Light pressure produces a wheal and flare formation with itching at the site of trauma within 5 min (Fig. 101). It may be associated with chronic urticaria but also occurs in around 5% of normal population.

Management

None may be required, or antihistamines.

Cholinergic urticaria

Clinical features

Common, predominantly affecting young adults and involving mainly trunk and limbs. Extremely itchy, micropapular, urticarial wheals occur in response to exercise, emotion or heat (Fig. 102).

Management

Antihistamines and anticholinergics may be helpful. Tends to resolve spontaneously.

Pressure urticaria

Clinical features

Rare; may be a component of ordinary chronic urticaria. Pressure produces painful swollen, indurated urticarial areas after several hours (Fig. 103). It may persist for 1–2 days.

Management

Cyproheptadine or other antihistamines can be tried, but the response is often disappointing. Oral steroids may be required.

Other physical urticarias

Clinical features

May be initiated by cold, heat, ultraviolet light, vibration and contact with water. Sometimes itching is the only feature.

Management

Antihistamines; avoidance of trigger factors; sunblocks for those reacting to light; advice on the dangers of swimming for those with cold or aquagenic urticaria.

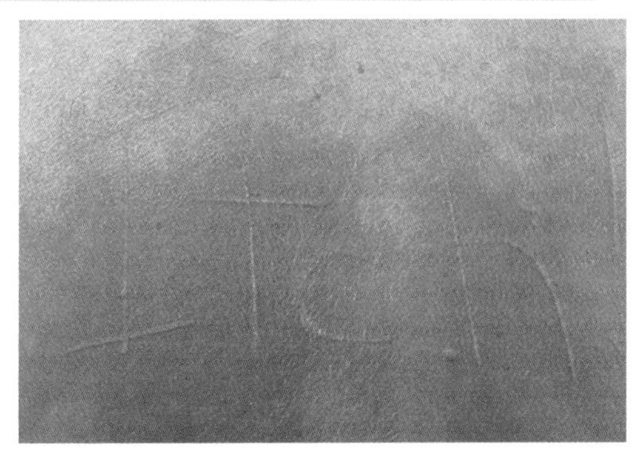

Fig. 101 Dermographism.

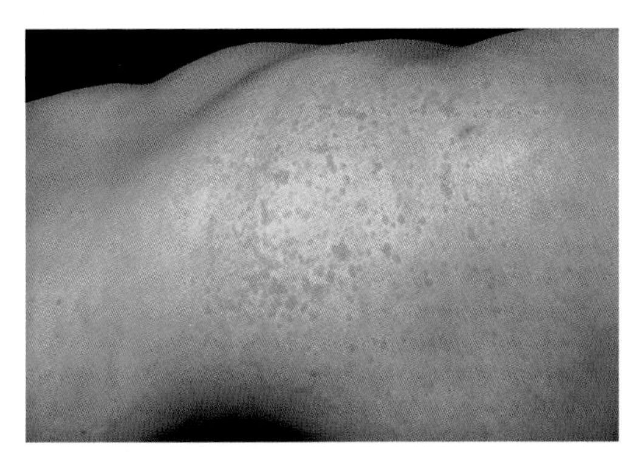

Fig. 102 Cholinergic urticaria.

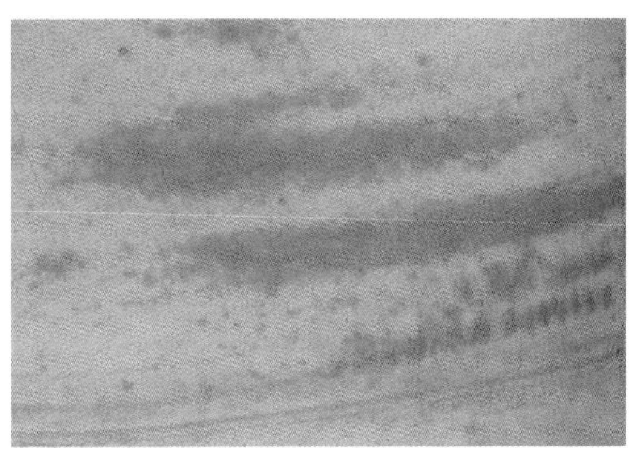

Fig. 103 Pressure urticaria from waistband.

18 Vasculitis

Erythema multiforme

Aetiology

A localized form of vasculitis. Attacks may be triggered by drugs and viral (especially herpes simplex) or *Mycoplasma* infections.

Clinical features

The eruption can occur at any age. There may be a prodromal illness. Initial lesions are dull, red, flat maculopapules spreading centrifugally, the centre becoming cyanotic, purpuric or even bullous or necrotic (Fig. 104). The characteristic target or iris lesions (Fig. 105) symmetrically involve the periphery (e.g. palms, dorsae of hands, feet, knees, elbows and forearms). Mucous membranes may be affected. A severe bullous form of erythema multiforme, Stevens–Johnson syndrome, with particular involvement of mucous membranes, can occur (Fig. 106). There is associated pyrexia and malaise, with oral, ocular and genital lesions. This form carries a significant morbidity and mortality.

Management

Usually symptomatic. Steroids may reduce the severity of attacks. The underlying cause should be removed or treated, where possible. Patients with severe recurrent erythema multiforme caused by herpes simplex may require treatment with continuous prophylactic aciclovir or by regular bimonthly injections of gammaglobulin.

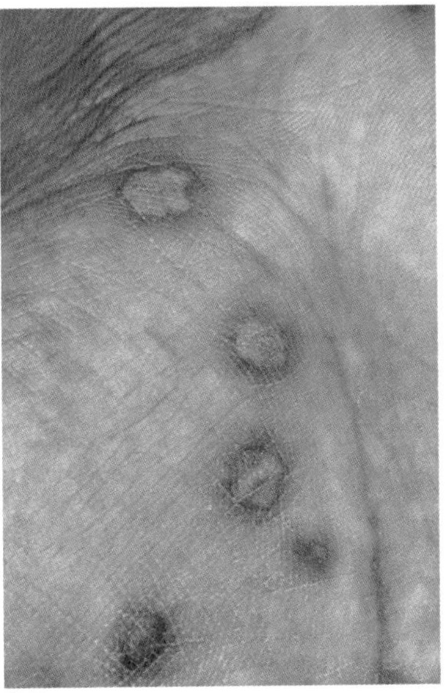

Fig. 104 Bullous erythema multiforme lesions of palm.

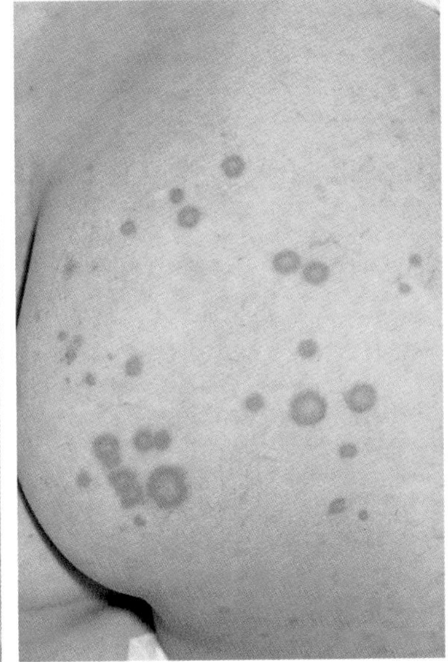

Fig. 105 Erythema multiforme: typical target or iris lesions.

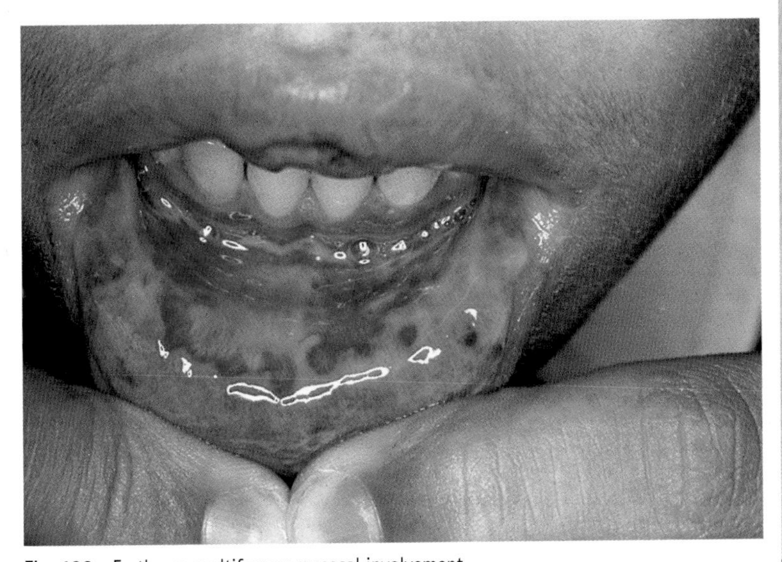

Fig. 106 Erythema multiforme: mucosal involvement.

Erythema nodosum

Aetiology

A common vasculitic reaction of larger subcutaneous vessels, due to a variety of provoking agents.

- Sarcoidosis
- Infections: streptococcus, tuberculosis, yersinia, infectious mononucleosis, virus, chlamydia
- Drugs: sulphonamides, oral contraceptives, salicylates, bromides or iodides, gold salts
- Inflammatory bowel disease

Clinical features

There may be a prodromal illness. Erythematous tender nodules appear on shins (Fig. 107) and occasionally thighs and forearms. There is associated pyrexia, malaise, oedema and aching of legs. The colour changes from bright red to purple to leave a brownish 'bruise'. Lesions occur in crops and recurrences may occur. Most attacks settle within 2–12 weeks.

Management

Bedrest, anti-inflammatory analgesics and support stockings or bandages. Systemic steroids may be required for severe cases.

Pyoderma gangrenosum

Aetiology

Unknown; often associated with diseases exhibiting altered or depressed immunity (e.g. leukaemias, myeloma, hyper- and hypoglobulinaemias, lymphoma). Other associations may include inflammatory bowel disease, rheumatoid arthritis, chronic active hepatitis, etc. Up to 30% of cases are idiopathic.

Clinical features

A destructive, necrotizing, inflammatory and vasculitic ulceration of the skin (Fig. 108). Initially presenting as furuncle-like nodule, pustule or haemorrhagic bulla. Toxicity, fever and leukocytosis occur in the acute phase.

Management

Treatment of underlying condition. High dose steroids initially. Ciclosporin and minocycline as alternatives.

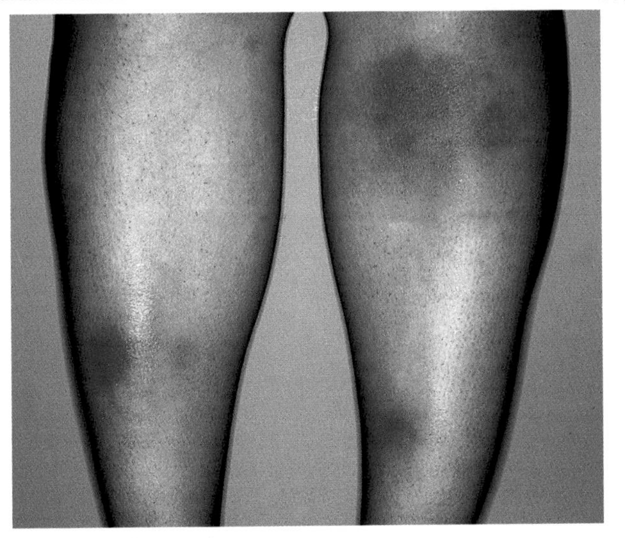

Fig. 107 Erythema nodosum.

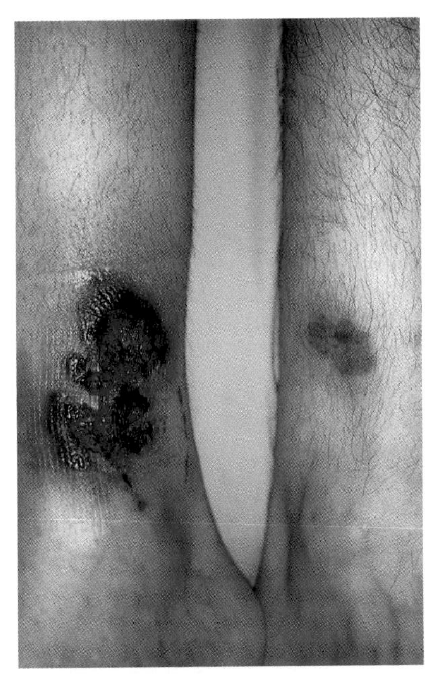

Fig. 108 Early lesions of pyoderma gangrenosum showing bluish undermined edges of ulcer.

Vasculitis

Aetiology

Immune complex deposition in blood vessels. Drugs, infections, ingested allergens and autoantigens have all been implicated.

Clinical features

Classically, the lower legs are affected, but the arms and trunk can also be involved (Fig. 109). Urticaria, toxic erythema and palpable purpura may progress to necrotic or bullous lesions (Fig. 110) with crusting and ulceration. Possible associated systemic vasculitis with renal, gastrointestinal and respiratory involvement and arthritis.

Management

Investigation of the underlying cause; bedrest. Systemic steroids may be required.

Capillaritis

Aetiology

Capillary leakage or vasculitis (Fig. 111). Most causes are cryptogenic (e.g. Schamberg's capillaritis), but some drugs produce a similar eruption. Stasis pigmentation also seen with venous hypertension or varicose veins (Fig. 112).

Clinical features

The idiopathic type usually affects the lower legs of young men. Discrete areas of asymptomatic red-brown, petechial or punctate purpura, becoming hyperpigmented.

Management

Support stockings may help.

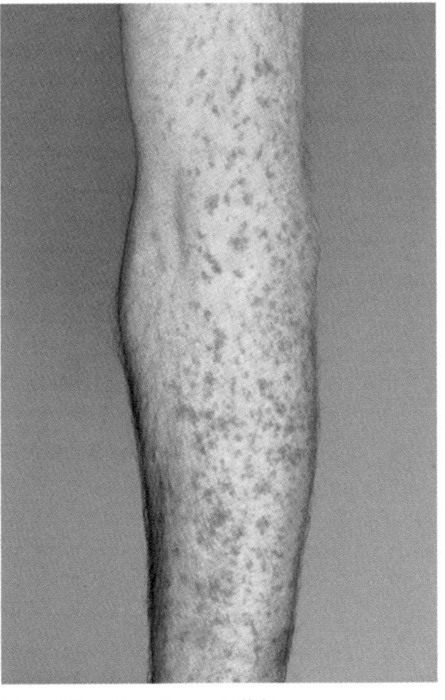

Fig. 109 Allergic vasculitis.

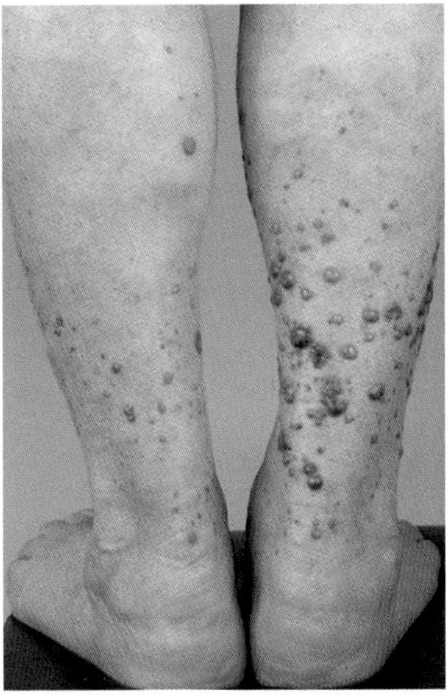

Fig. 110 Leukocytoclastic vasculitis.

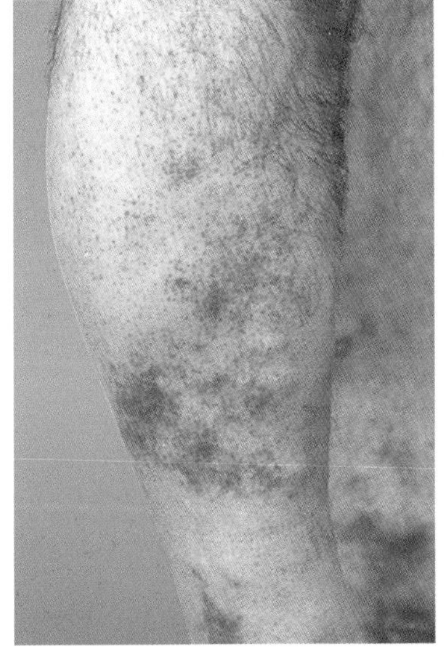

Fig. 111 Capillaritis with 'cayenne pepper' pigmentation.

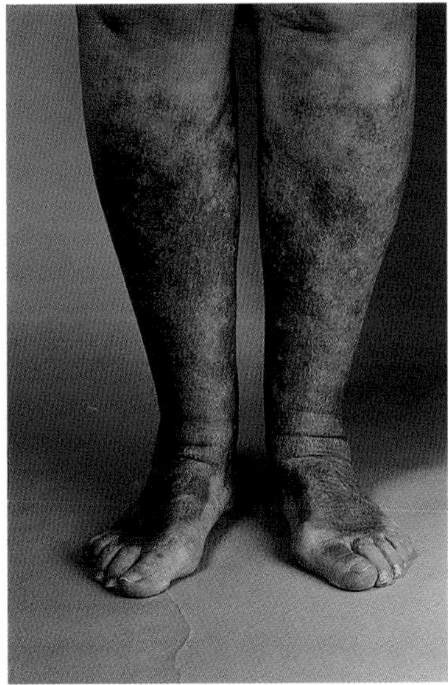

Fig. 112 Stasis pigmentation.

19 Leg ulcers

Stasis eczema and venous ulceration

Aetiology

Venous hypertension results from deep vein thrombosis or familial valvular incompetence, with incompetent or perforating veins leading to poor tissue perfusion and the development of stasis eczema (Fig. 113) and ulcers (Fig. 114).

Clinical features

Usually seen in obese, middle aged women, with characteristic inverted 'champagne bottle' leg. Skin changes usually start on the medial aspect of lower leg at site of perforating veins, as stasis pigmentation or lipodermatosclerosis. There is often oedema or lymphoedema (elephantiasis nostras) (Fig. 115); or the leg may become progressively more fibrotic and sclerotic (Fig. 116), with strangled microcirculation (atrophie blanche) and cutaneous ischaemia.

Complications

Ulceration can often follow minimal trauma with the 'atrophie blanche' type leg. Secondary infection is invariable, but normally only pathogenic bacteria (group A streptococci and *Staphyloccus aureus*) require treatment. Streptococcal infection may cause cellulitis. Topical antibiotics frequently provoke allergic contact sensitization (Fig. 123, p. 77).

Management

Weight reduction; compressive or 4-layer bandaging or short stretch bandaging; support stockings when ulcers are healed; rest with legs up. Oil helps scaly dry skin. Antiseptic solutions can be used to clean ulcers before applying simple dressings (e.g. paraffin gauze, povidone-iodine, bio-occlusive or hydrocolloid dressings). Systemic antibiotics can be administered for clinical infection; moderate strength steroid ointments for eczema. Surgery may be required for varicosities or incompetent perforators.

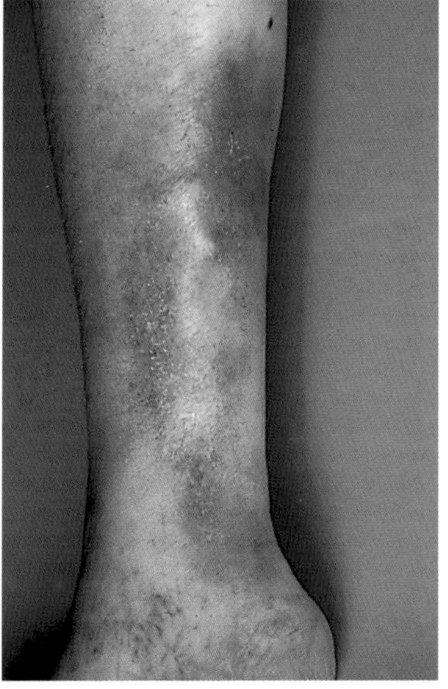

Fig. 113 Incompetent perforating vein with associated stasis eczema and lipodermatosclerosis.

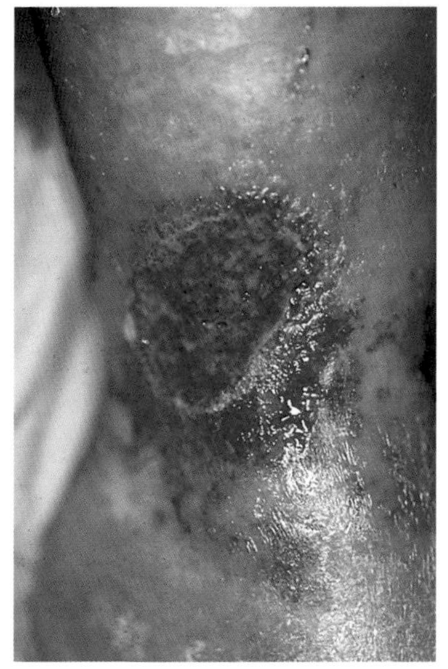

Fig. 114 Venous ulcer.

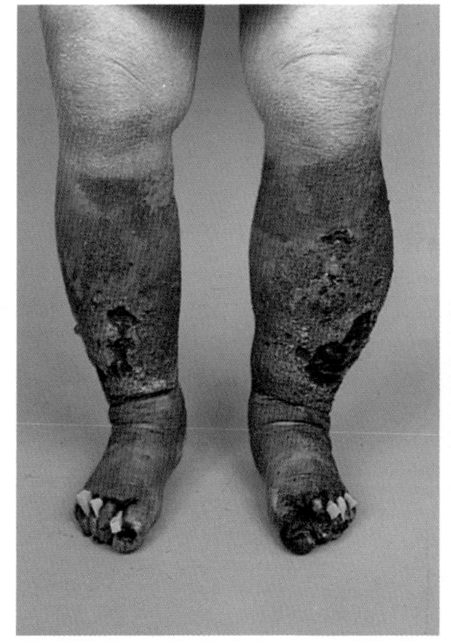

Fig. 115 Elephantiasis nostras.

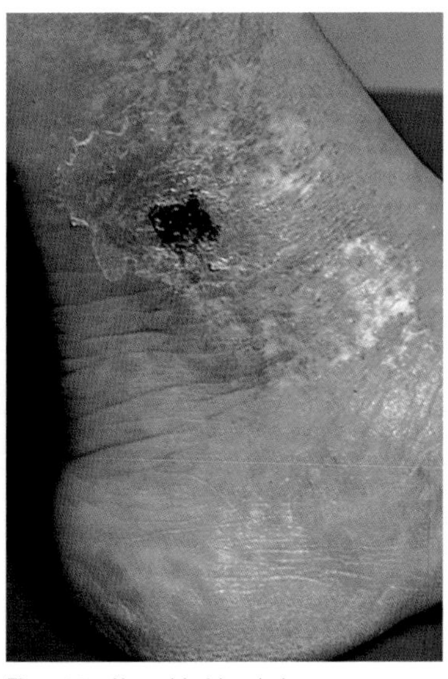

Fig. 116 'Atrophie blanche'.

Leg ulcers

Aetiology

- Secondary to venous hypertension (p. 72).
- Secondary to arterial disease. Ulceration may follow arterial thrombosis, atherosclerosis, vasculitis or small vessel disease, such as that associated with rheumatoid arthritis and diabetes. Hypertension is an important complicating factor.
- Neuropathic ulcers occur in diabetics (Fig. 117), alcoholics, and patients with Hansen's disease (leprosy). They particularly involve the foot or lower leg. Secondary infection also often plays a part.
- Malignancy—a progressive, non-healing or 'atypical' leg ulcer should raise the question of a basal cell or squamous cell carcinoma.
- Other rare causes include sickle cell disease, spherocytosis, cryoglobulinaemia and tertiary syphilis (Fig. 118).

Clinical features

Venous ulcers Often large and messy, and usually associated with other signs of venous hypertension (p. 72).

Arterial ulcers More often affect the foot and lateral aspects of the legs. Peripheral pulses may be diminished or absent, and pain is a constant feature, especially at night or when dressings are too tight. The ulcers have a characteristic 'punched out' appearance (Fig. 119) with a well-defined regular edge.

Management

Treatment of venous ulcers is discussed on page 72. In arterial disease, treatment is generally unsatisfactory since the underlying cause of the ischaemia is rarely reversible. Hypertension should be controlled. (NB: beta-blockers reduce tissue perfusion.) Appropriate antibiotics should be used for secondary infection; intravascular abnormalities should be corrected where possible. Adequate analgesia is important, and dressings should be simple and non-constricting. In some cases vascular reconstruction may be possible; in other cases chemical sympathectomy, epoprostenol infusions or pentoxifylline may give relief.

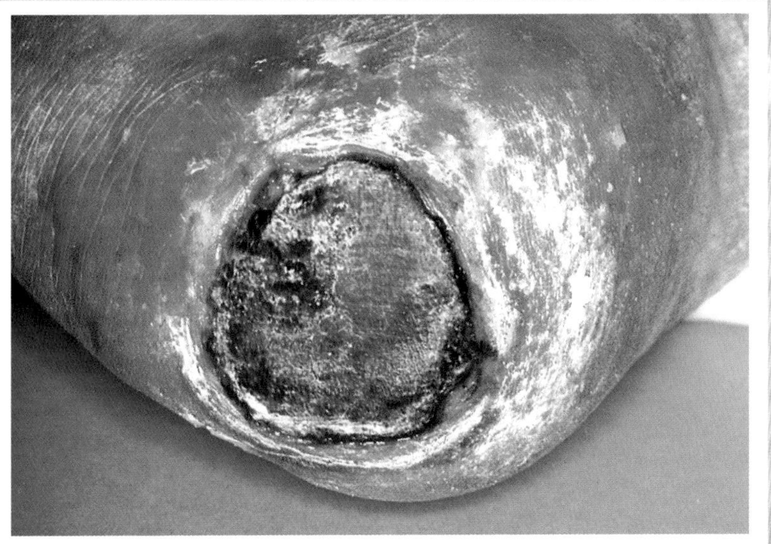

Fig. 117 Ischaemic neuropathic or pressure ulcer on heel of diabetic patient.

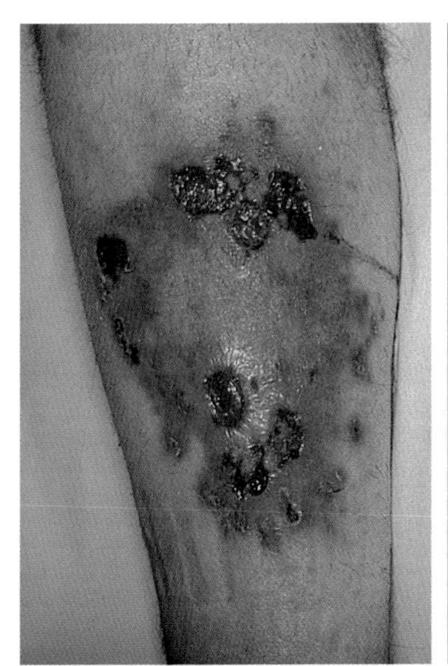

Fig. 118 Atypical ulceration (syphilis).

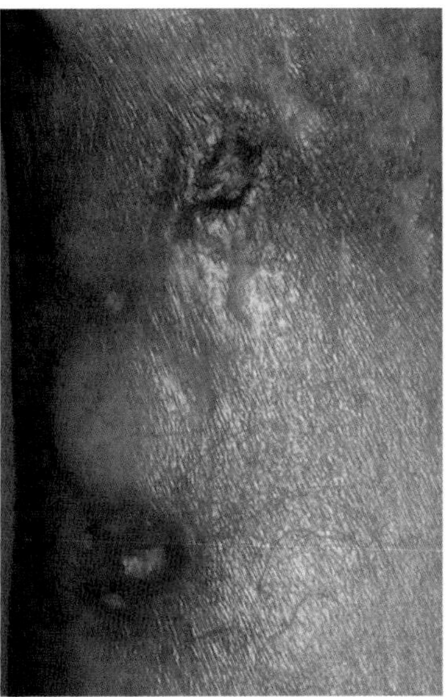

Fig. 119 Small punched out arterial ulcers.

20 Contact dermatitis

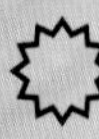

Aetiology

Irritant contact dermatitis (ICD) May be acute (strong irritants) or cumulative (mild irritants—e.g. detergents/solvents), with progression from irritant reaction (dryness/chapping) to dermatitis. Atopy is a predisposing factor.

Allergic CD (Figs 120–123) Due to type IV (delayed) lymphocyte-mediated hypersensitivity. Common allergens include nickel, chromate, rubber chemicals, medicaments and cosmetics (preservatives, fragrance). Industrial allergens include epoxy, acrylate and phenol formaldehyde resins. Plant allergens include Compositae (chrysanthemums, dandelions, asters, etc.), *Primula obconica*, Rhus (poison oak, poison ivy) and various other woods and balsams.

Photo CD May be allergic (e.g. sunscreens), toxic (phytophotodermatitis) or light-aggravated (Compositae plants).

Clinical features

Hands and face, being in most contact with the environment, are the sites most commonly affected. The cause of the dermatitis may be obvious from the history, but patch testing is often necessary. Facial allergens may be volatile (airborne) or cosmetic. Medicament CD may be a complicating factor in stasis ulcers, chronic ear and eye disorders and pruritus ani or pruritus vulvae due to prolonged usage on damaged skin.

Management

Identify cause and advise on avoidance or protection. Soap substitute (e.g. aqueous cream) can be used to clean or wash; 'barrier' creams make hands easier to clean but afford no protection. Other treatments include emollients, topical steroids in strengths appropriate to severity of eczema and, rarely, systemic steroids. Antihistamines are not particularly helpful.

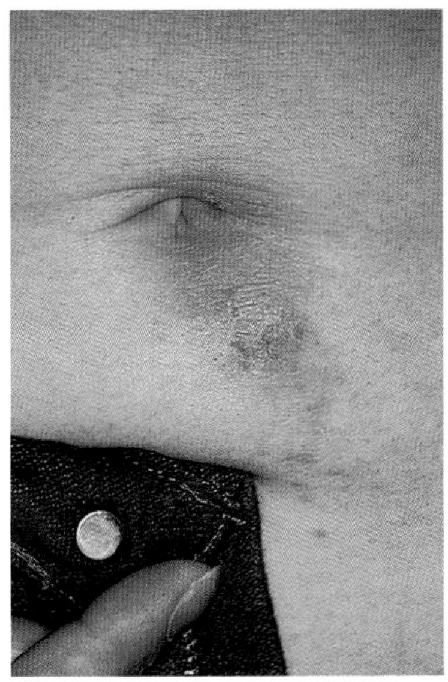

Fig. 120 Allergic contact dermatitis due to nickel jean stud.

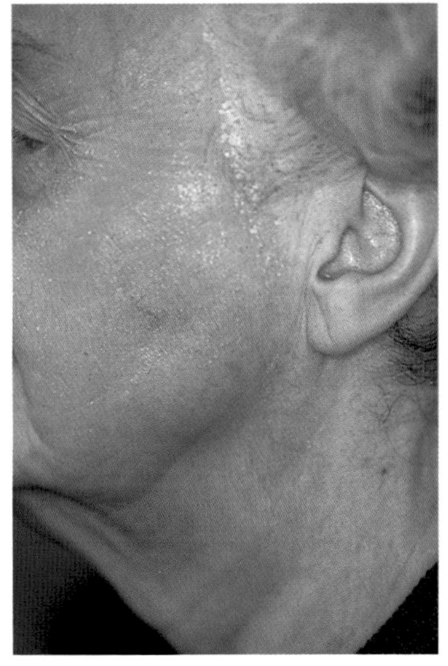

Fig. 121 Volatile type of allergic contact dermatitis due to phosphorus sesquisulphide in matches.

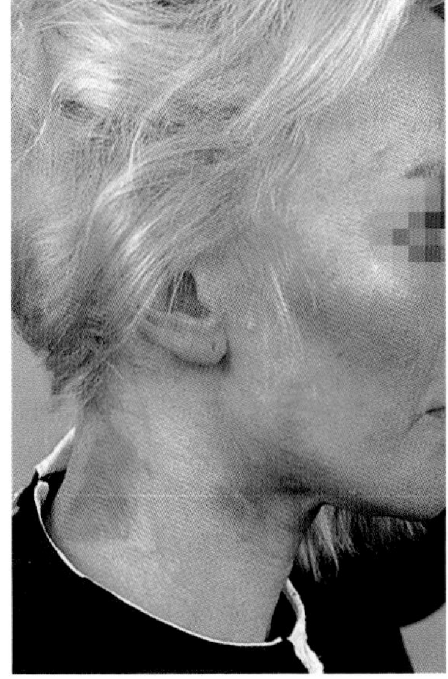

Fig. 122 Patchy erythema on neck due to nail varnish.

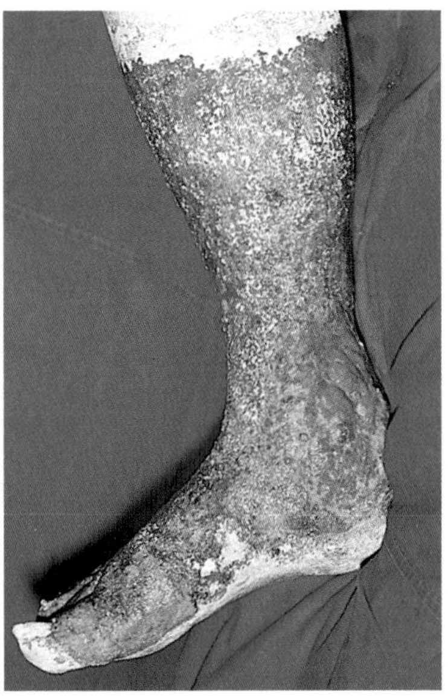

Fig. 123 Lower leg is an important site for medicament sensitivity.

21 Hand eczema

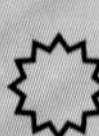

Synonym
Hand dermatitis.

Aetiology
Constitutional or exogenous, or frequently both, and impossible to differentiate on clinical appearances alone (Fig. 124). Atopic persons are more prone to irritant hand eczema.

Clinical features
Constitutional patterns (p. 80) Include recurrent pompholyx; vesiculo-squamous; vesicular-hyperkeratotic and hyperkeratotic.

Exogenous patterns include

1. Irritant patterns
   - 'Ring' eczema from wet work and detergents (Fig. 125).
   - 'Web' eczema on dorsum of hands from wet work.
   - 'Finger-tip' and 'palmar' patterns due to wet cloths, frictional factors, etc.
   - 'Patchy' or 'discoid' patterns.
2. Allergic patterns
   - 'Non-specific'. Most cases (e.g. from perfumes, preservatives, etc.) will be missed unless routine patch testing is performed.
   - 'Specific patterns' (e.g. rubber glove dermatitis) (Fig. 126), ring dermatitis and fingertip eczema.
   - Atopic individuals, especially those who are health care workers, may also develop type I contact urticaria to natural rubber latex, and those who are food handlers may develop contact urticaria or protein contact dermatitis to foods.

Management
Identify the cause. Patch testing is helpful. Provide hand care advice (e.g. cotton-lined PVC gloves for wet work and frequent applications of emollients). Potent steroids, with antibiotics for secondary infection. Atopic persons with a history of eczema should be given employment counselling.

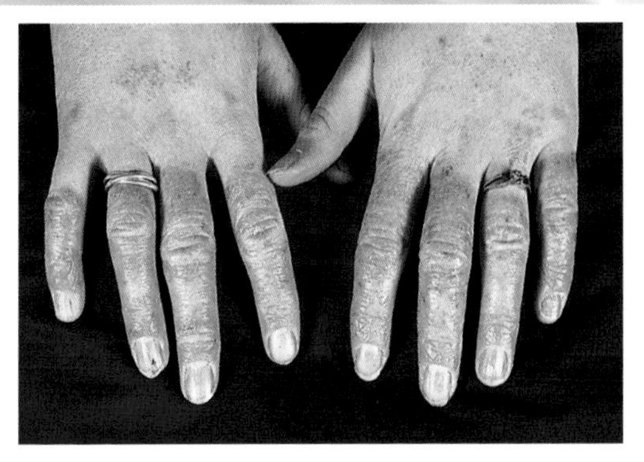

Fig. 124 Hand dermatitis: irritant and allergic factors frequently coexist.

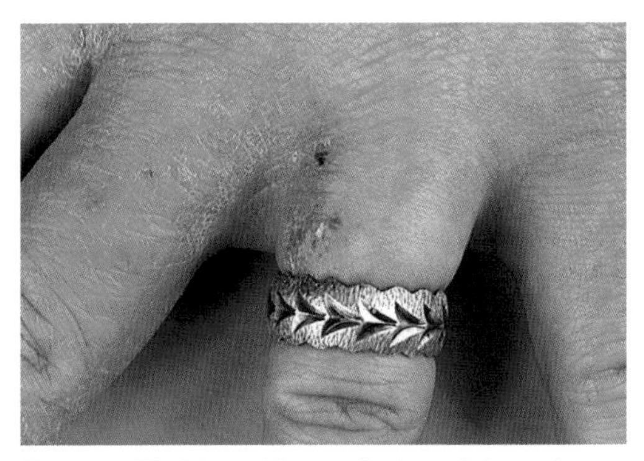

Fig. 125 'Ring' dermatitis—may be due to irritants, but occasionally is associated with nickel allergy.

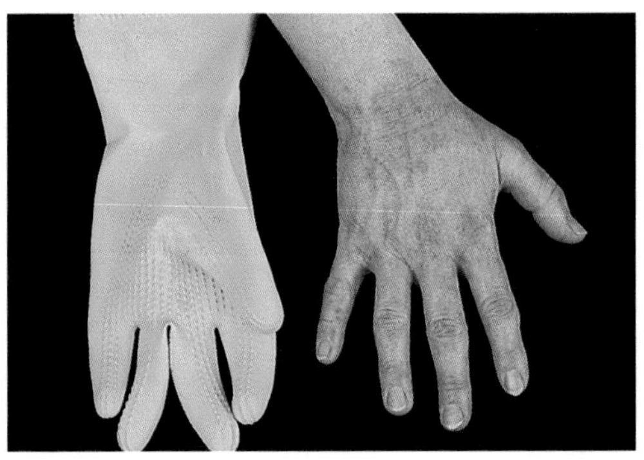

Fig. 126 Allergic contact dermatitis due to rubber gloves.

Pompholyx

Aetiology

A common form of endogenous eczema. It may be a reaction to an active fungal infection of the feet. Ingested allergens (e.g. nickel in females) are sometimes implicated. Most cases are cryptogenic or constitutional.

Clinical features

A recurrent, intensely itchy, symmetrical eruption of the hands (with or without the feet) with crops of clear vesicles on the sides of fingers and palms (Fig. 127). These may become confluent, producing large bullae (Fig. 128). Secondary infection is common. Skin subsequently becomes dry or fissured and desquamates. In Europe the more chronic relapsing form of vesiculo-squamous palmar eczema is also known as dyshidrotic eczema.

Management

- Frequent potassium permanganate (1:8000) or acetic acid/aluminium acetate soaks initially.
- Potent topical steroids or steroid/antibacterial combinations.
- Sedating antihistamines for symptomatic relief.
- Systemic steroids for severe attacks.
- Oral antibiotics if secondary infection is present.
- Treat athlete's foot if present.

Hyperkeratotic palmar eczema

Aetiology

Uncommon pattern of constitutional eczema not related to atopy. Factors include friction and underlying hyperkeratotic or psoriasiform tendency.

Clinical features

Usually affects middle-aged adults, with intensely itchy, hyperkeratotic patches of fissured eczema on palms (Fig. 129). Rarely, there may be a few vesicles.

Management

Potent topical steroids, antipruritic antihistamines, soap substitutes/emollients, tar, avoidance of friction, keratolytics or acitretin if hyperkeratosis severe; low dose systemic steroids or other immunosuppressants or superficial radiotherapy (rarely) for intractable disease.

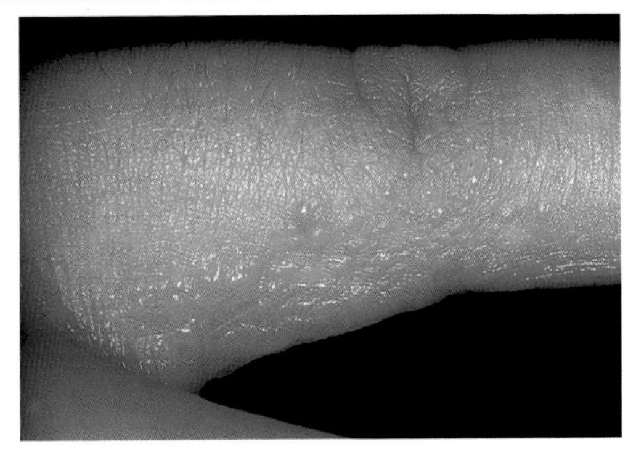

Fig. 127 Vesicular hand dermatitis (pompholyx).

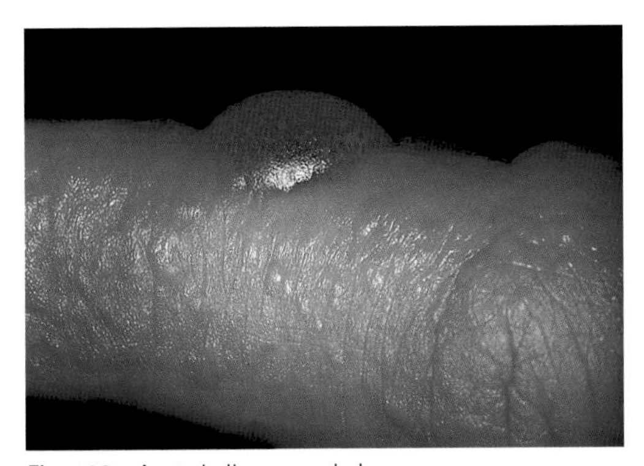

Fig. 128 Acute bullous pompholyx.

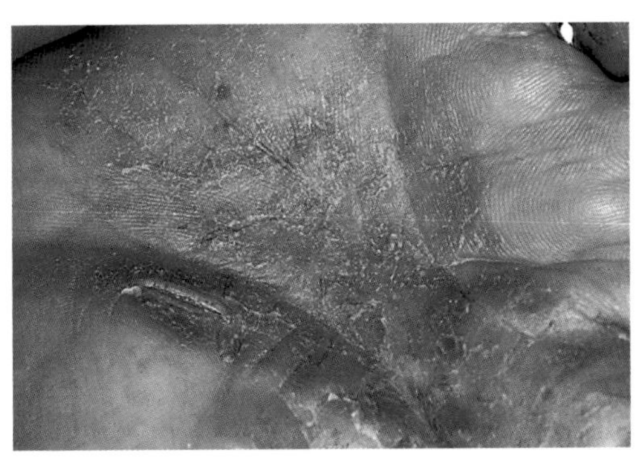

Fig. 129 Hyperkeratotic hand eczema.

Other eczemas

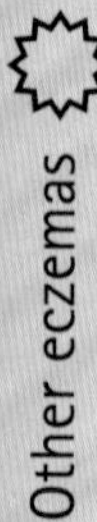

Seborrhoeic eczema

Aetiology

Unknown. *Pityrosporum ovale* or *P. orbiculare* infection may be important.

Clinical features

Infantile 'Cradle cap' (p. 14); napkin (p. 12).

Adult In young adults (usually men), it commonly involves scalp, ears, eyebrows, eyelids, nasolabial folds, central chest and pubic area (Figs 130–132). There are greasy scales on a background of erythema associated with generally greasy, easily irritated or intolerant skin. This is a chronic relapsing condition, and flares are often associated with stress. In the elderly, involvement is commonly intertriginous. Moist erythematous areas are often the sites of secondary bacterial (or candidal) infection.

Management

Soap substitutes; weak topical steroids, steroid/imidazole combinations; sulphur and salicylic acid creams and tar or imidazole shampoos; steroid scalp applications.

Asteatotic eczema

Aetiology

Reduced lipids and water binding capacity of the stratum corneum leads to drying or cracking of the skin. The condition is aggravated by excess washing and low temperature or humidity. It is occasionally associated with malnutrition, general debility, diuretic therapy, myxoedema and renal failure.

Clinical features

Common in middle to old age; itchy, dry and scaly with reticulate cracks (Fig. 133). Normally affects legs, but trunk and arms may be involved. Rarely, there may be an underlying malignancy.

Management

Emollients, bath oils, fewer baths; weak topical steroid ointments.

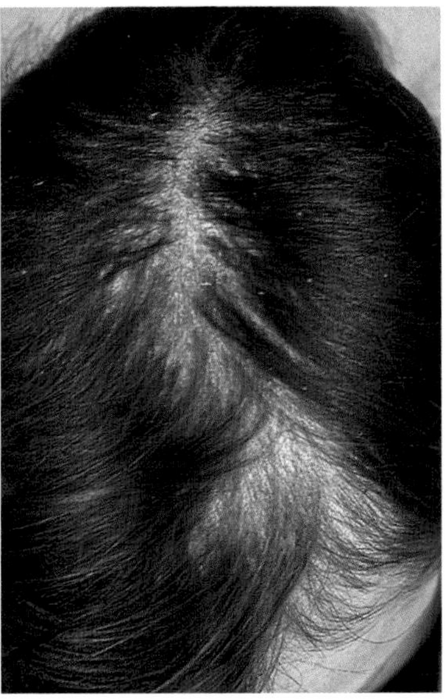

Fig. 130 Seborrhoeic dermatitis of scalp.

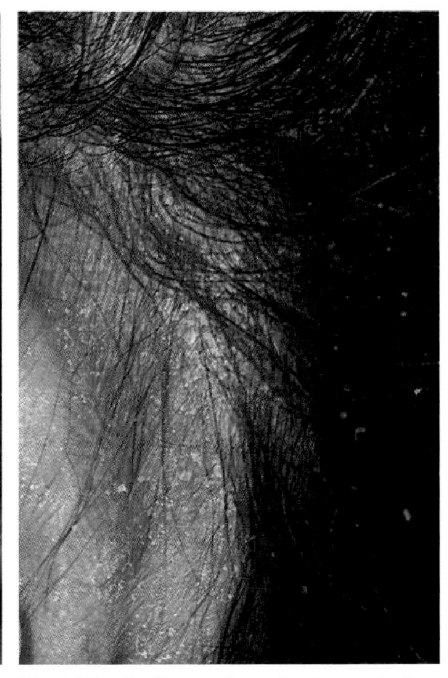

Fig. 131 Scalp margin and retro-auricular seborrhoeic dermatitis.

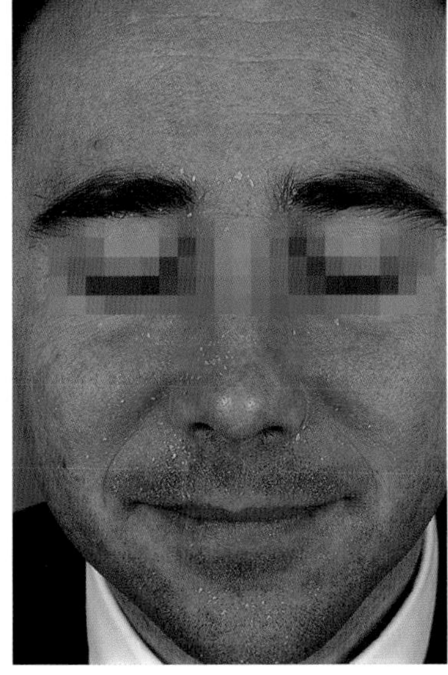

Fig. 132 Characteristic facial seborrhoeic dermatitis.

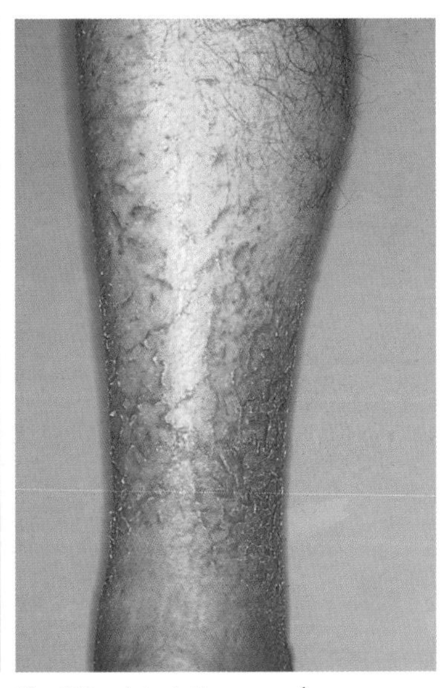

Fig. 133 Asteatotic eczema (eczema craquelé).

Discoid eczema

Synonym

Nummular eczema.

Aetiology

A constitutional pattern of eczema. The condition characteristically occurs in middle-aged men (executives), and stress, over-washing and low humidity (e.g. central heating, air-conditioning, car heaters, etc.) may be important.

Clinical features

Well-demarcated coin-shaped areas of eczema (Fig. 134) normally affect the extensor surfaces of limbs (Fig. 135), but with subsequent explosive spread to a more generalized pattern of eczema (Fig. 136). One or two solitary patches often predate the general eruption by some weeks or months. Pruritus may be intense. Lesions are often vesicular and exudative and may become secondarily infected. Discoid eczema may sometimes be associated with an 'extensor' pattern of atopic eczema and, rarely, with contact allergy (e.g. chromate). Initially often mistaken for fungal infection.

Management

Soap substitutes; a reduction in bathing; an increase in the humidity of surroundings. Treatments also include emollients, sedative oral antihistamines, potent steroids or steroid/antibacterial combinations and oral antibiotics. Systemic steroids may sometimes be required, and tar may be of help in more chronic cases.

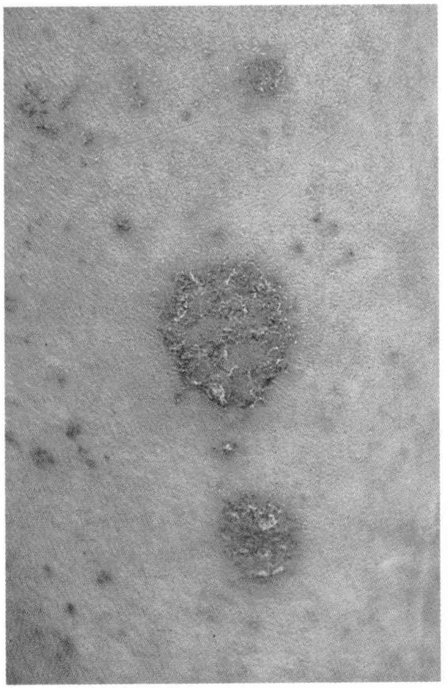

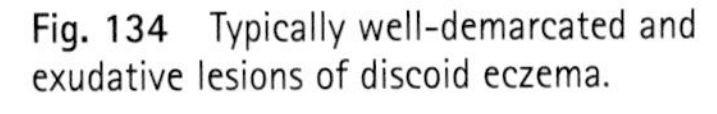

Fig. 134 Typically well-demarcated and exudative lesions of discoid eczema.

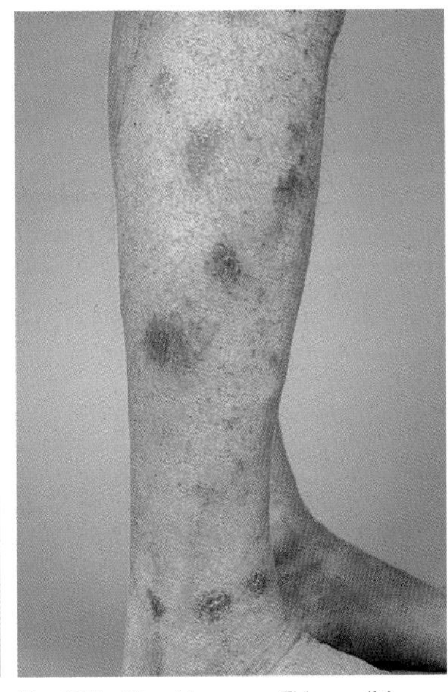

Fig. 135 Discoid eczema. This condition may sometimes be mistaken for a fungal infection.

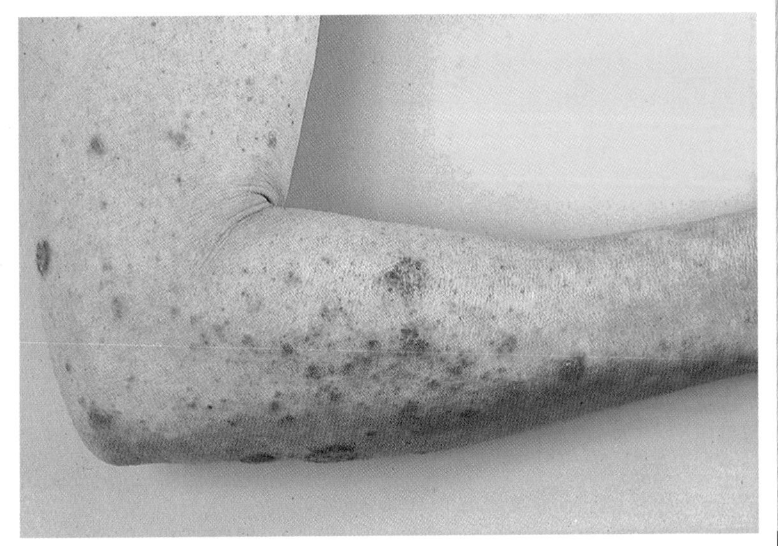

Fig. 136 Discoid eczema with secondary spread.

23 Localized patterns of itch

Lichen simplex (neurodermatitis)

Aetiology

A localized, sometimes eczematous response to constant rubbing; often partly habit and frequently triggered by stress.

Clinical features

Several characteristic patterns:

- Women—nape of neck, side of neck, front of elbow and vulva.
- Men—ankle or shin (Fig. 137), scrotum and perianal area (Figs 138, 139).
- Both sexes—central palms and ears (otitis externa).

The lichenified lesions are either solitary and well demarcated or more diffuse, as on the scrotum and perianal area, due to repeated scratching and rubbing (Fig. 140).

Management

Potent topical steroids (only mild to moderate strength for perineal lesions), tar paste bandages or occlusion with bio-occlusive dressings, sedative antihistamines, occasionally intralesional steroids. Habit reversal and cognitive therapy.

Pruritus ani

Aetiology

Predisposing factors include haemorrhoids, fissures, irritation from mucous or faecal leak, sweat or maceration, contact dermatitis, threadworm infection (in children).

Clinical features

Lichen simplex, maceration, fissuring or bacterial/candidal intertrigo (Fig. 139).

Management

Treat underlying or complicating factors. Soap substitutes, mild to moderate corticosteroid/antimicrobial preparations; sedative antihistamines. Risk of secondary contact dermatitis.

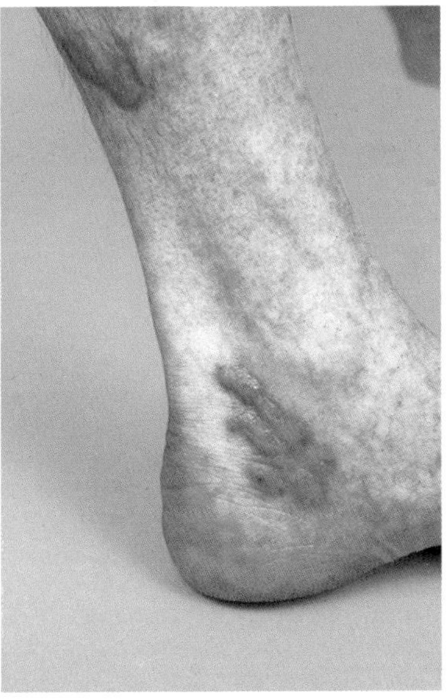

Fig. 137 Lichen simplex chronicus.

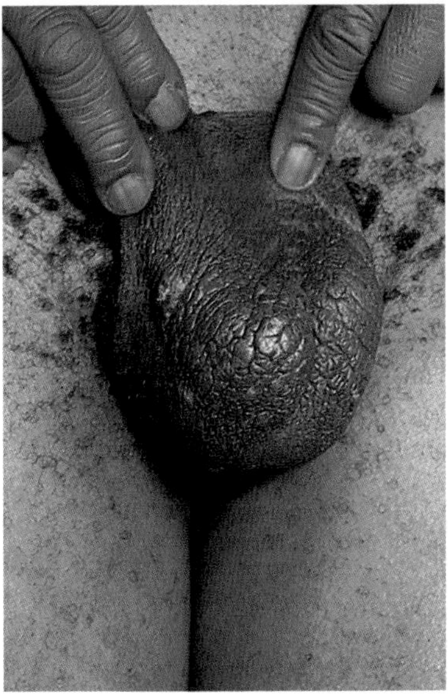

Fig. 138 Lichen simplex of scrotum.

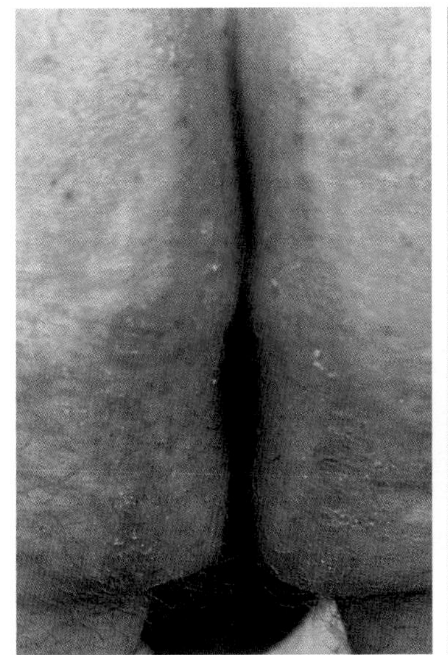

Fig. 139 Pruritus ani/perianal dermatitis.

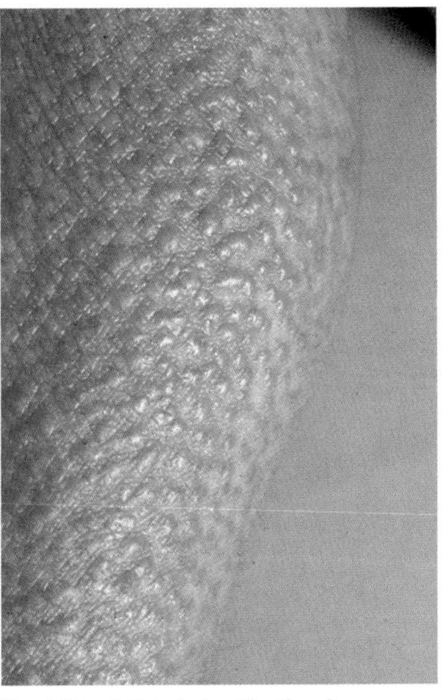

Fig. 140 Pebbly lichenification from constant rubbing.

Prurigo

Clinical features

'Prurigo' is a term used to describe any localized skin abnormality in which the principal symptom is itch. Lesions include excoriations, prurigo nodules and localized areas of lichen simplex.

'Cape prurigo' A common pattern in the elderly (Fig. 141). Dry skin and low serum iron concentrations are important factors.

'Tycoon scalp' (Fig. 142) A characteristic pattern of excoriation of the scalp, mainly affecting businessmen and frequently associated with stress. Folliculitis and seborrhoeic dermatitis may be initiating factors.

Subacute prurigo Mainly affects the extensor aspects of limbs in women, but more diffuse patterns also occur.

Nodular prurigo An intransigent pattern of prurigo with intensely pruriginous nodules separated by areas of normal skin. It mainly affects the extensor aspects of limbs (Fig. 143).

Management

'Cape prurigo' often responds to simple emollients, iron replacement therapy and sedative antihistamines. Weak steroid creams may also be helpful. Thyroid disease and pre-pemphigoid need to be excluded. Other patterns of prurigo are very intransigent and respond poorly to treatment. The itch-scratch-itch habit is difficult to break. Potent steroids, occlusive tar paste bandages or bio-occlusive dressings, sedative antihistamines, phototherapy and, occasionally, intralesional steroids are required. Cognitive therapy and habit reversal techniques may also help.

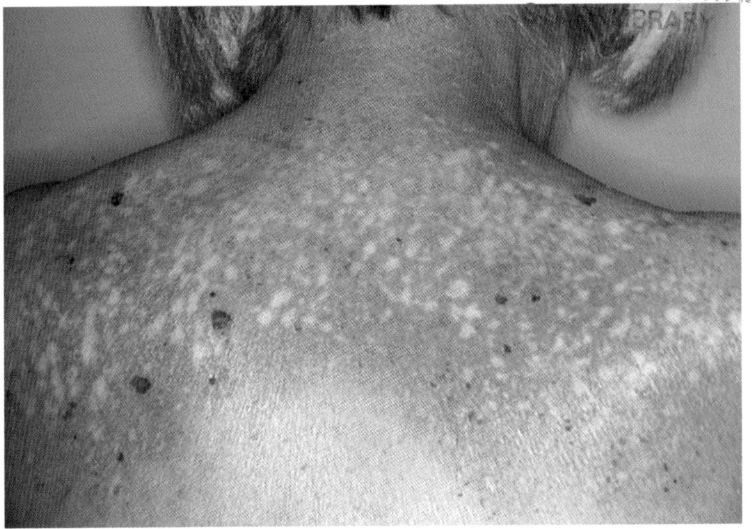

Fig. 141 'Cape prurigo': a common manifestation of iron deficiency in the elderly.

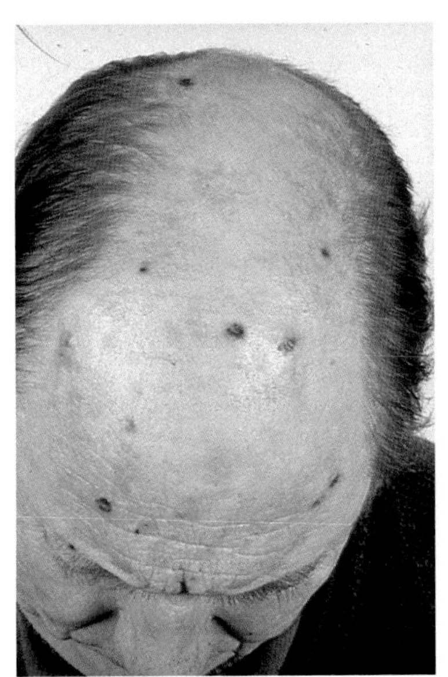

Fig. 142 Tycoon scalp.

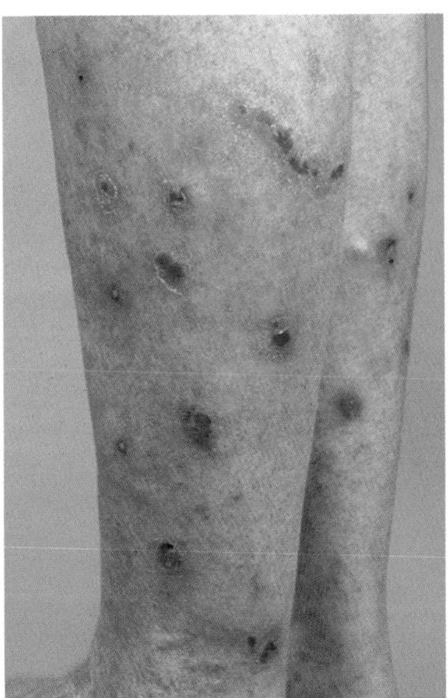

Fig. 143 Nodular prurigo.

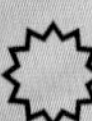

Vitiligo

Aetiology

One of a group of organ-specific autoimmune diseases with anti-melanocyte antibodies.

Clinical features

Well-defined oval or irregular depigmented areas (symmetrical and a few mm to several cm in size) affecting axillae, groins, genitalia, dorsum of hands and face (Figs 144 & 145). Hair in the affected areas may also become white. The involved skin tends to burn on sun exposure but is otherwise asymptomatic. Other organ-specific autoimmune diseases may coexist (e.g. thyroid disease, pernicious anaemia, diabetes mellitus and alopecia areata) in both patients and their families (Fig. 146).

Management

Not universally successful. Repigmentation may sometimes be induced with intermittent phototherapy or potent topical steroids. Cosmetic camouflage is helpful (taught by Red Cross cosmetic camouflage teams). Sunscreens are essential both to prevent burning of the depigmented areas and to reduce tanning in normal areas. Micrografts are also successful in some patients.

Halo naevus

Aetiology

Localized form of vitiligo.

Clinical features

An area of depigmentation surrounding a small pigmented cellular naevus (Fig. 147). The central naevus usually disappears over several months, and repigmentation may then occur, or a leukodermic area may persist. Some patients develop vitiligo.

Management

Sunscreens to protect vitiliginous area.

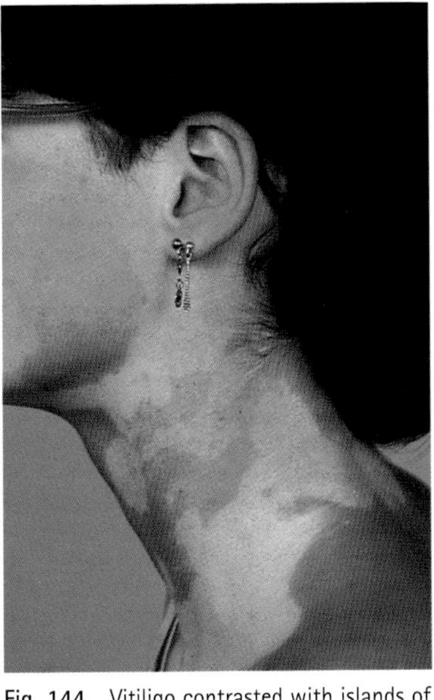

Fig. 144 Vitiligo contrasted with islands of normally pigmented skin.

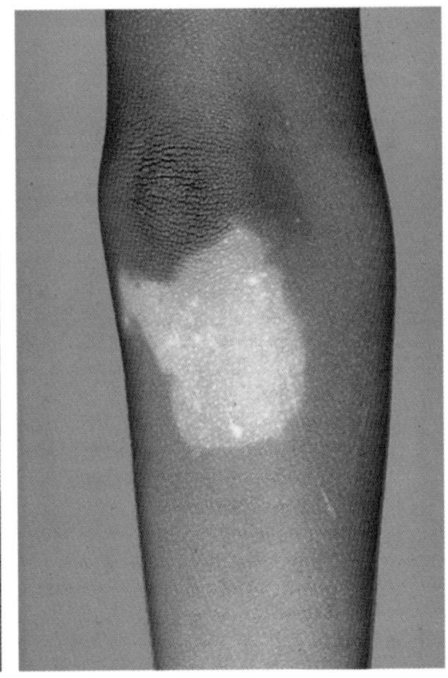

Fig. 145 Vitiligo in a dark-skinned girl.

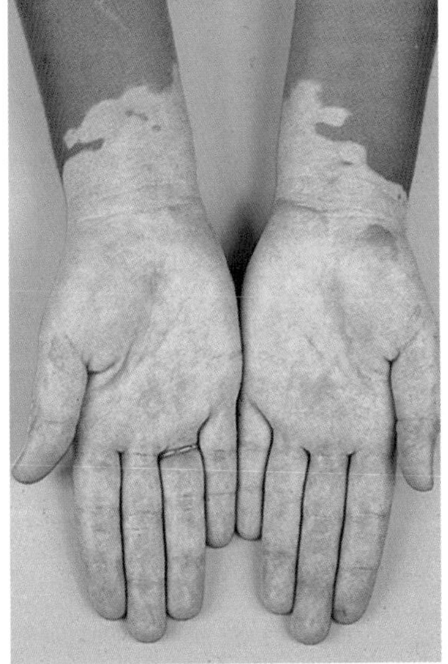

Fig. 146 Vitiligo in a patient with co-existent Addison's disease.

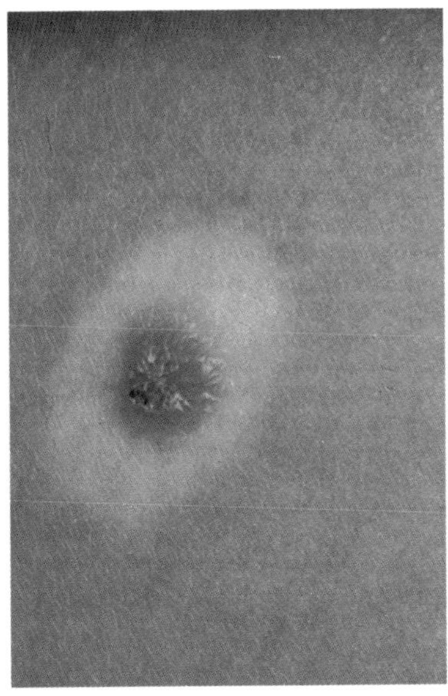

Fig. 147 Halo naevus.

Scleroderma

Synonym

Systemic sclerosis; acrosclerosis; morphoea.

Aetiology

Unknown but thought to be autoimmune.

Clinical features

There are three principal types of scleroderma.

- A multisystem disease (acrosclerosis) commonly affects women. Raynaud's phenomenon is a frequent presenting symptom. Skin of the hands and face is hard and tightly bound down. Fingers become tapered, flexed, shiny with loss of finger pulps (sclerodactyly) (Fig. 148). There may be nail fold thromboses and fingertip ulceration. Telangiectasia and calcium deposits in the fingers are common. The gastrointestinal tract, liver, kidneys, joints and lungs may also be involved.
- A more progressive form (progressive systemic sclerosis) affects both sexes equally. Morbidity and mortality are significant.
- Localized cutaneous scleroderma (morphoea) normally affects young adults, women more than men. Ill-defined purplish, sclerotic plaques develop insidiously, usually on the trunk, and progress slowly over months to years.

Management

Always very disappointing. Calcium channel blockers for Raynaud's phenomenon. Localized morphoea may resolve spontaneously.

Dermatomyositis

Aetiology

Unknown, possibly autoimmune, sometimes paraneoplastic (underlying malignancy or lymphoma).

Clinical features

Affects skin, muscles and blood vessels. Characteristic heliotrope erythema and oedema of face or exposed sites (Fig. 149) associated with muscle weakness and inflammation. Raynaud's phenomenon, nail fold telangiectasia (Fig. 150), photosensitivity and calcinosis may coexist. Creatine phosphokinase (CPK) levels are often raised.

Management

Oral steroids with or without azathioprine. Bedrest initially. Occasionally other immunosuppressants, intravenous immunoglobulin, physiotherapy, sunscreens.

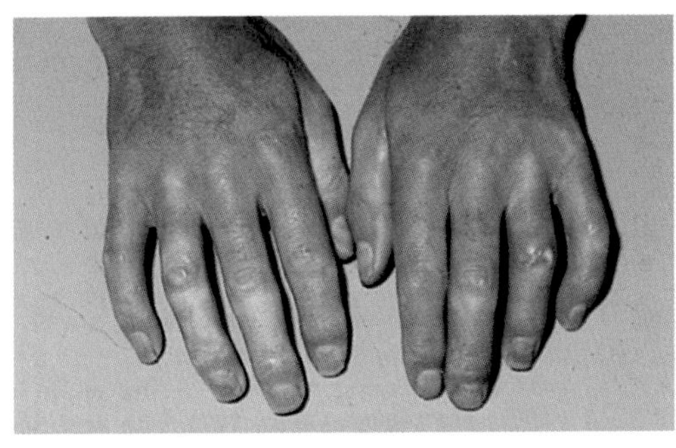

Fig. 148 Acrosclerosis.

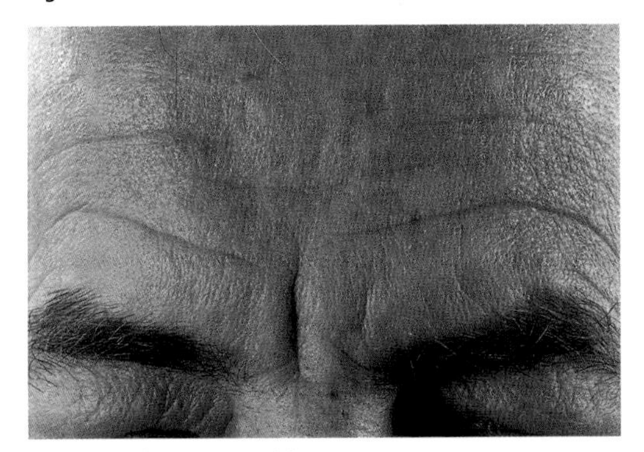

Fig. 149 Dermatomyositis.

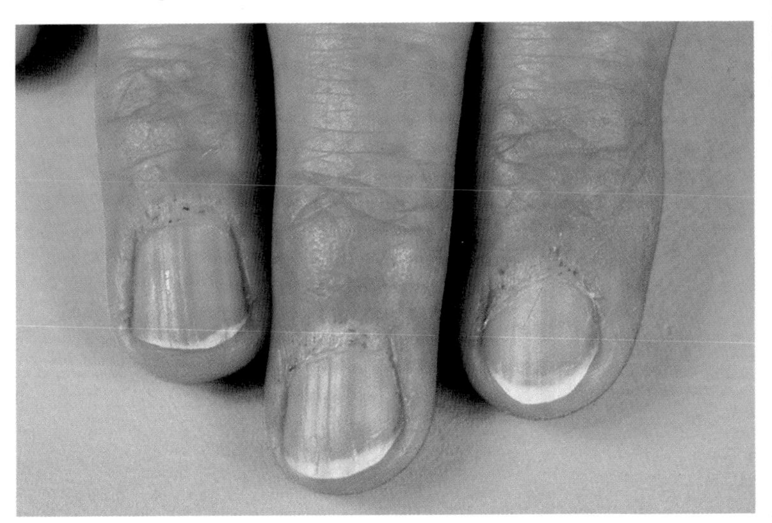

Fig. 150 Nail fold thromboses in a patient with dermatomyositis.

25 Lichen planus

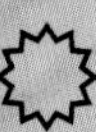

Aetiology

Unknown, although an autoimmune basis is likely.

Clinical features

The characteristic skin lesions are small, itchy, shiny, flat-topped, violaceous papules (Fig. 151) with an overlying network of fine white lines (Wickham's striae) (Fig. 152). The eruption usually affects the wrists, forearms and trunk, lasting from 6 months to 2 years. The buccal and genital mucosae are also often affected with typical milky, 'lace-like' streaks or violaceous or atrophic patches. Mucosal patches may progress to superficial erosive lesions that are particularly painful on the perineum and heal with scarring. Scalp involvement may produce scarring alopecia, and permanent nail loss may occur if nail involvement is severe. Lesions occurring on the shins tend to coalesce and produce hypertrophic plaques (Fig. 153). Fading skin papules leave post-inflammatory hyperpigmentation. Lichen planus may also occur at sites of trauma (Fig. 154). This is known as the Köbner phenomenon and is also seen in psoriasis, in vitiligo and with certain viral infections such as molluscum contagiosum and plane warts.

Management

Topical steroids and sedative antihistamines are helpful for symptomatic relief, although in mild cases no treatment may be required. Hypertrophic plaques can be treated with potent topical steroids or injected with intralesional steroids. There are also several proprietary steroid and anti-inflammatory agents that can be used for the mouth. Potent steroids are needed for perineal lesions to try to reduce scarring.

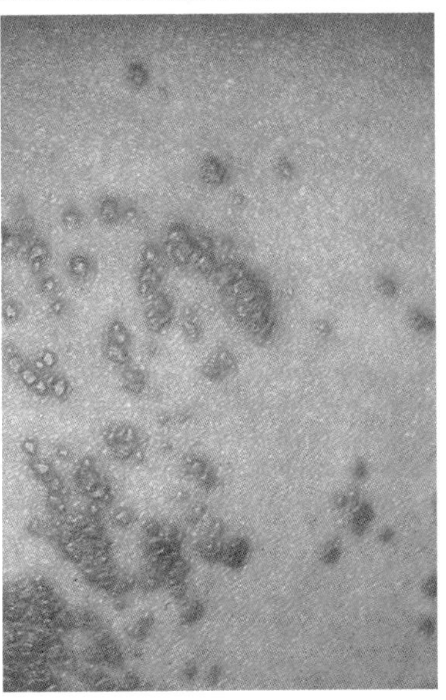

Fig. 151 Flat-topped violaceous papules of lichen planus.

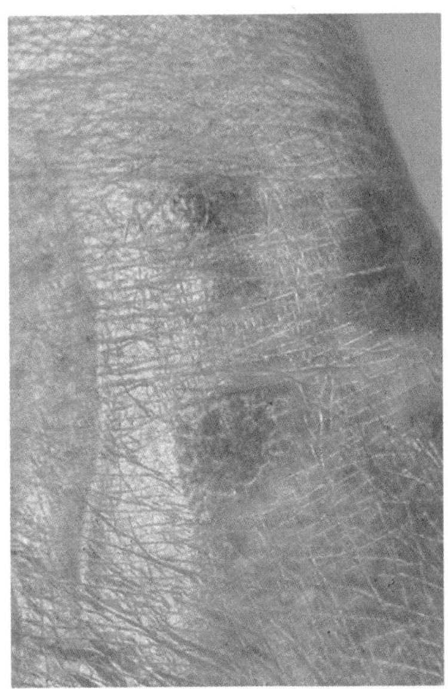

Fig. 152 Wickham's striae (lichen planus).

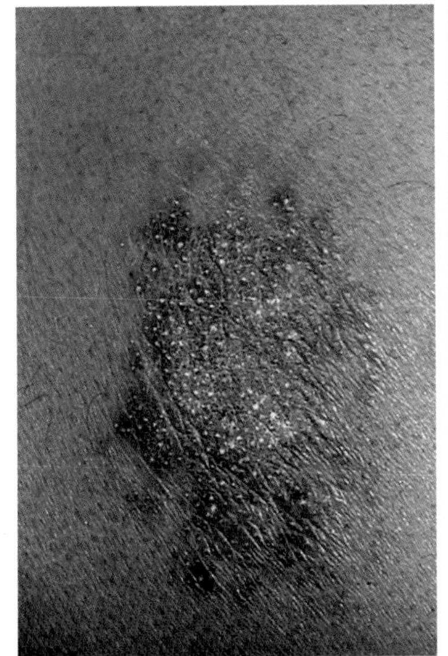

Fig. 153 Hypertrophic lichen planus.

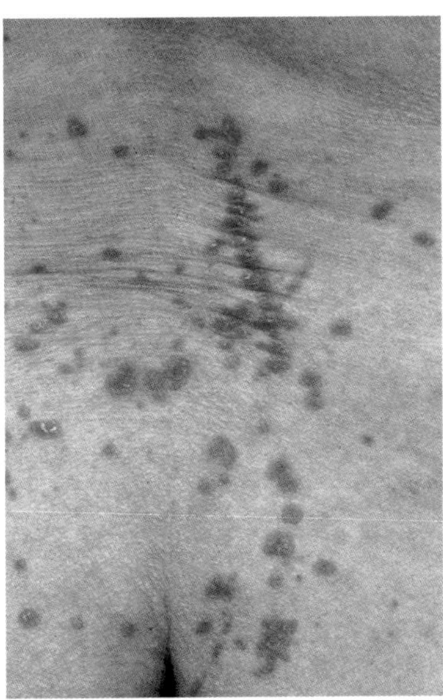

Fig. 154 Lichen planus (Köbner phenomenon).

26 Lupus erythematosus (LE)

Discoid (cutaneous) lupus erythematosus (DLE)

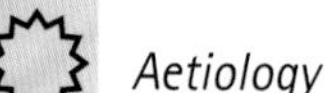

Aetiology
Autoimmune disorder.

Clinical features
Symmetrical, well-defined plaques of erythema with scaling, atrophy and follicular plugging (Fig. 155). It mainly affects light-exposed areas, such as face, (Fig. 156) neck, scalp, ears, upper chest, back and backs of hands and is frequently exacerbated by sunlight. Scalp involvement may produce scarring alopecia.

Management
Avoidance of sunlight. Sunscreens, topical steroids and hydroxychloroquine may be required.

Systemic lupus erythematosus (SLE)

Aetiology
Autoimmune. Genetic predisposition. Pregnancy may act as a trigger. Drugs can sometimes provoke an SLE-like syndrome.

Clinical features
A multisystem disease affecting women more frequently than men. The skin, joints, kidneys, lungs, central nervous system and other organs may all be involved. Lymphopenia and thrombocytopenia are common. There is often an element of photosensitivity or an eruption confined to light-exposed areas. This may be 'discoid LE–like', non-specific erythema or a maculopapular eruption. The classic pattern consists of a symmetrical patchy erythema, sometimes with scaling, telangiectasia and induration, occurring on the cheeks and bridge of the nose producing a typical 'butterfly' rash (Fig. 157). The hands are often affected, and there may be vasculitis (p. 70), livedo and chilblain-like lesions during the winter (Fig. 158). Nail fold infarcts and splinter haemorrhages with Raynaud's phenomenon may be present (p. 92). There may be general symptoms, including arthralgia, malaise and fever. Alopecia occurs in up to 50% of patients.

Management
Avoidance of exacerbating factors (e.g. cold and sunshine). Systemic steroids and immunosuppressants are usually required for more severe disease. Monitor renal function.

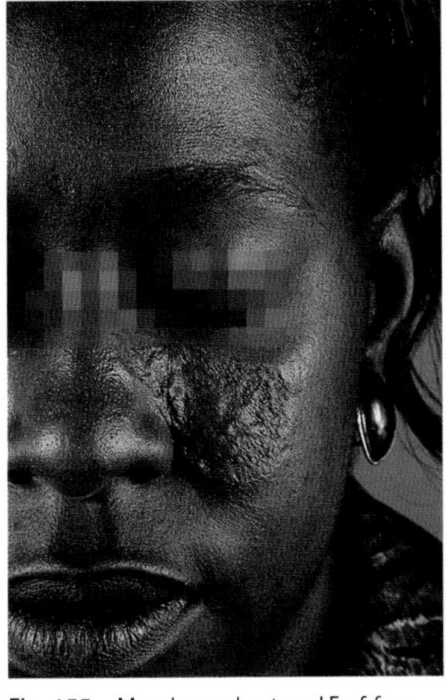

Fig. 155 Maculopapular-type LE of face.

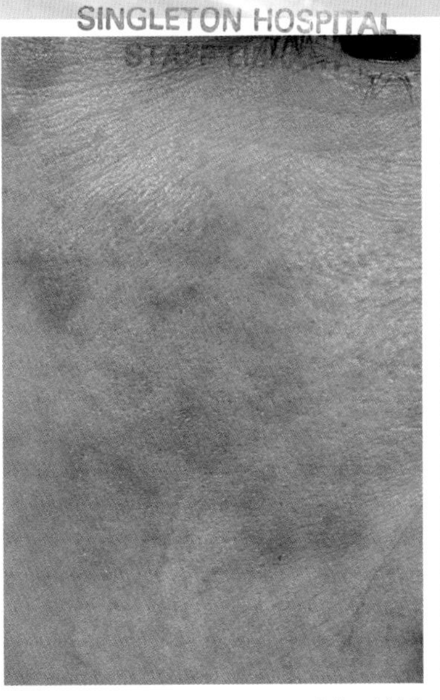

Fig. 156 Well-defined plaque of discoid LE with follicular plugging and scarring and post-inflammatory pigmentation.

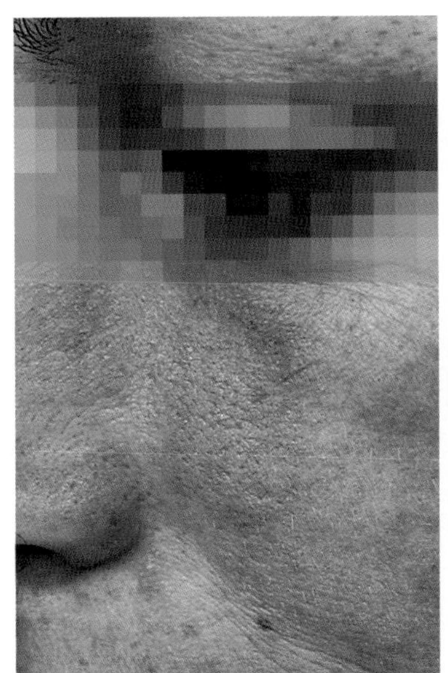

Fig. 157 Classic 'butterfly' rash of LE.

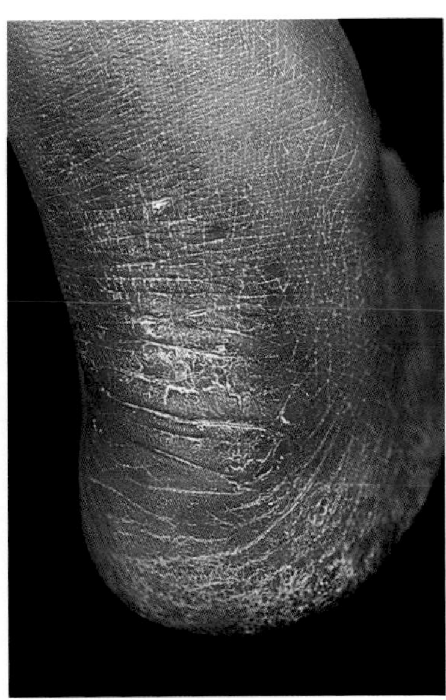

Fig. 158 'Chilblain' LE.

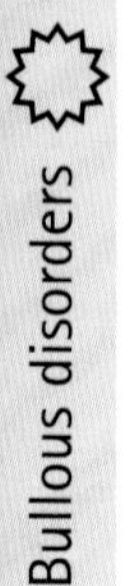

Dermatitis herpetiformis

Aetiology

Autoimmune disease associated with gluten enteropathy and immunoglobulin A (IgA) deposits in the skin.

Clinical features

Groups of small blisters or papulovesicles on an urticated background often starting on elbows (Fig. 159) and involving elbows, knees, buttocks, scalp and scapular areas. Intensely itchy excoriations rather than blisters are usually seen (Fig. 160).

Management

Can be controlled by dapsone. A strict gluten-free diet is necessary.

Pemphigus

Aetiology

Autoimmune disease directed against epidermal cells and intraepidermal components.

Clinical features

A disease of the middle-aged. Widespread, erythematous erosions (or true blisters that rupture very easily) can occur on any area of the body (Fig. 161). Firm pressure on the surrounding skin will produce a sore (Nikolsky sign). Mucous membranes are also involved. Tends to be fatal if left untreated.

Management

High doses of systemic steroids initially; azathioprine as a steroid-sparing agent. Other immunosuppressives/cytotoxics sometimes required.

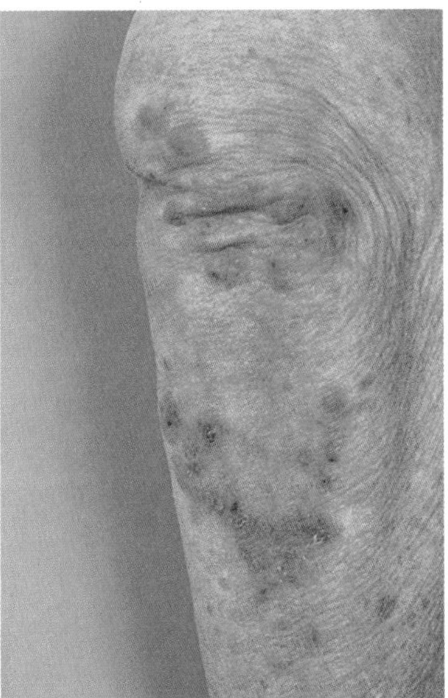

Fig. 159 The elbows are a characteristic site of involvement in dermatitis herpetiformis.

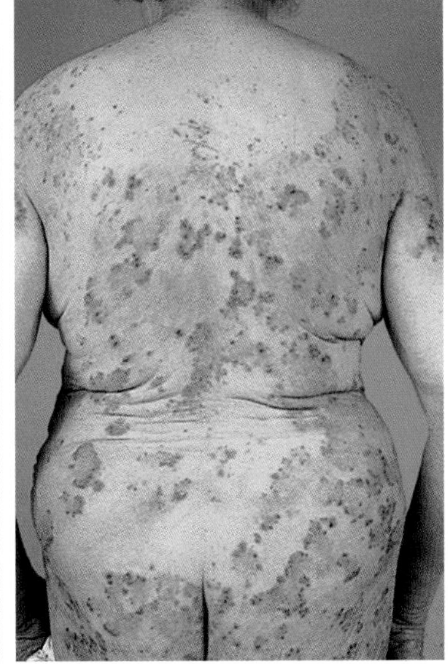

Fig. 160 Urticarial and annular lesions in dermatitis herpetiformis

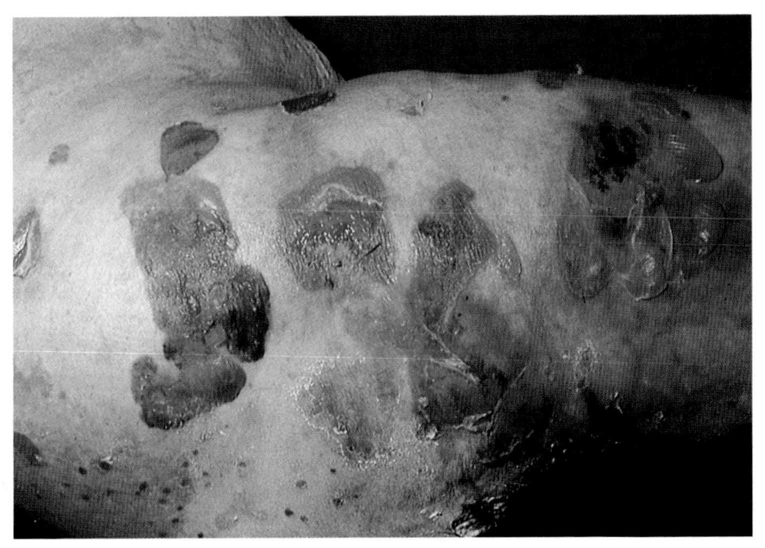

Fig. 161 Flaccid blisters and erosions in pemphigus.

Pemphigoid

Aetiology

Autoimmune disease directed against the basement membrane of the skin.

Clinical features

A disease of the elderly. An urticated eruption develops initially often on the limbs (Fig. 162). Irritation is usually intense. Blisters usually appear within a few days, are large, thick-walled and tense and do not rupture easily (Fig. 163). Disease soon becomes widespread and symmetrical. Mucosal involvement is relatively uncommon.

Management

High doses of systemic steroids initially; lower maintenance dose for several months. Azathioprine or other cytotoxics/immunosuppressants may be used as steroid-sparing agents. Dapsone and potent topical steroids may be effective for mild or localized disease. Tetracyclines and nicotinamide are also sometimes effective.

Cicatricial (mucosal) pemphigoid

Aetiology

Autoimmune disease closely related to pemphigoid.

Clinical features

A disease of the elderly. Blisters rupture to produce superficial erosions, which heal with scarring. The mucous membranes of the mouth and conjunctivae are most frequently affected (Fig. 164), but the nose, throat, genitalia, anus and oesophagus can be involved. Scarring causes adhesions between conjunctival surfaces and scarring alopecia on the scalp.

Management

As for pemphigoid. Ocular involvement must be treated by an ophthalmologist.

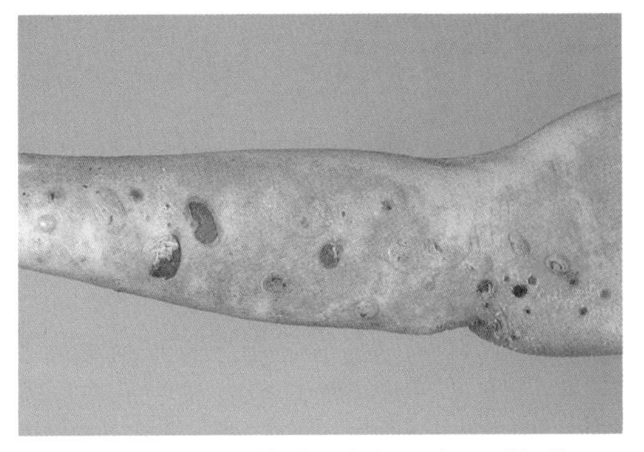

Fig. 162 Urticated and bullous lesions of pemphigoid.

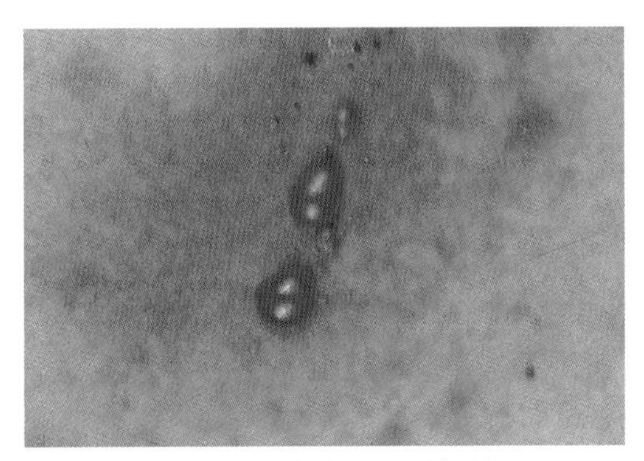

Fig. 163 Tense blisters in bullous pemphigoid.

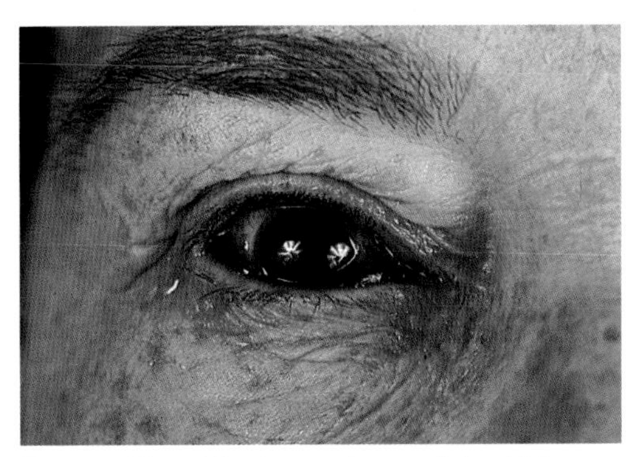

Fig. 164 Mucosal involvement in case of cicatricial pemphigoid.

28 Drug reactions/eruptions

The wide availability and use of drugs makes a drug history extremely important.

Aetiology

Hypersensitivity reactions can occur where the drug or drug metabolite acts as an antigen. However, many eruptions remain idiosyncratic.

Clinical features

Urticarial (p. 60), eczematous, bullous and lichenoid reactions may be seen. Other eruption patterns include the following.

Morbilliform Common maculopapular pattern of drug eruption, which mimics viral exanthems. A good example of this is the ampicillin rash in patients with glandular fever. Other antibiotics and phenothiazines may give a similar reaction pattern (Fig. 165).

Vasculitis Produced by many drugs, including sulphonamides (see p. 66).

Erythema multiforme/Stevens–Johnson syndrome Typical target lesions may be caused by barbiturates, phenytoin, gold, phenylbutazone and sulphonamides. Severe cases can progress to Stevens–Johnson syndrome with severe mucosal involvement (Fig. 166).

Purpuric Drugs can produce purpura (Fig. 167) by direct capillary damage or via thrombocytopenia (e.g. gold salts, quinine, quinidine, thiazides and benzodiazepines).

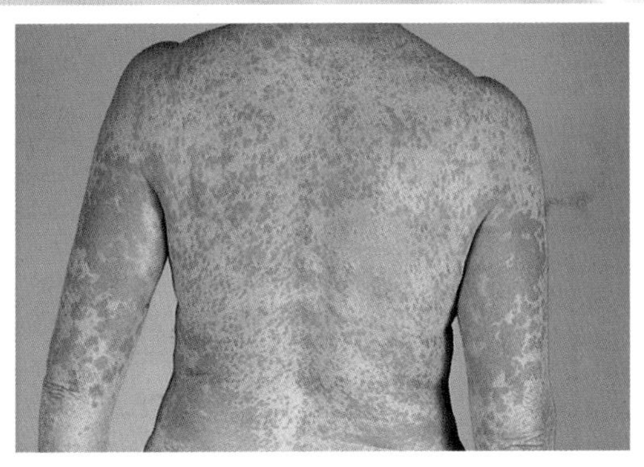

Fig. 165 Morbilliform 'ampicillin'-type rash.

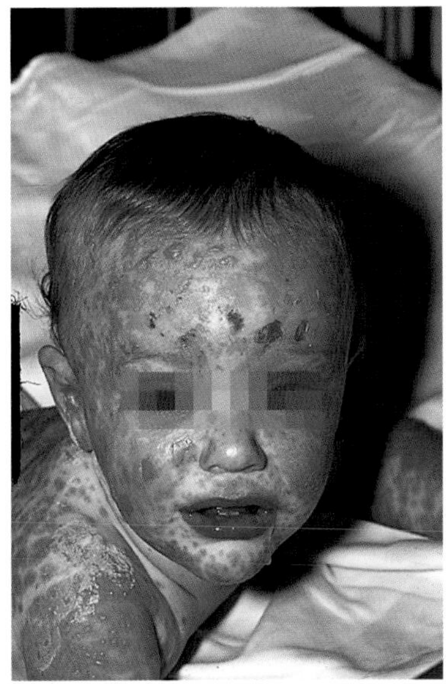

Fig. 166 Stevens–Johnson syndrome.

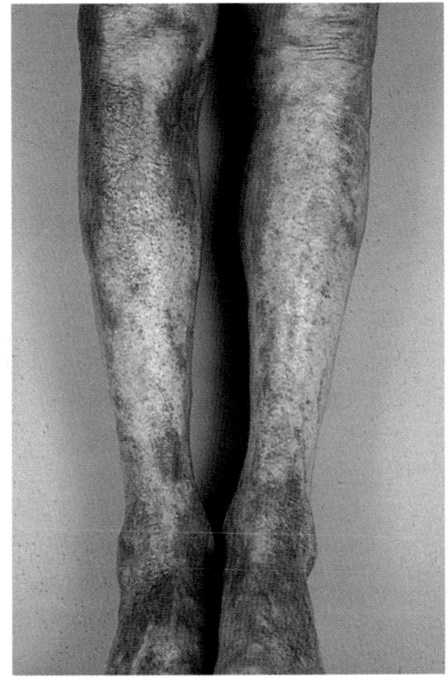

Fig. 167 Purpuric drug rash.

Toxic epidermal necrolysis Large areas of epidermis are lost, leaving extensive denuded areas of skin (p. 18). Fluid loss, electrolyte imbalance and secondary infection are frequent complications. The condition has a significant mortality and may be caused by various drugs, including barbiturates, sulphonamides, phenytoin, phenylbutazone and other NSAIDs.

Fixed drug eruption These lesions are characteristically well demarcated and dusky red, often with central blistering (Fig. 168) and subsequent post-inflammatory pigmentation. The eruption occurs at the same sites each time the drug responsible is taken, although new sites may also be affected. Mucosal lesions are common. Laxatives containing phenolphthalein, barbiturates and sulphonamides are common offenders.

Photosensitivity Phototoxic reactions can occur with drugs that would not usually produce a skin eruption without sun exposure (p. 36). The distribution is typical, being confined to exposed areas (e.g. face, arms and 'V' of neck). Shaded areas such as those under the chin and ears are often spared. Photoallergic reactions can also occur. Thiazides, sulphonamides, chlorpromazine, tetracyclines and nalidixic acid may all be responsible.

Pigmentation Pigmentation may occur with some drugs, especially amiodarone (Fig. 169), phenothiazines, phenytoin, chloroquine, mepacrine, busulfan or other cytotoxic drugs, clofazimine and minocycline. Melasma (Fig. 171) develops in constitutionally predisposed individuals due to exposure to sunshine and endogenous (pregnancy) or exogenous oestrogens and progestogens (e.g. oral contraceptives).

Erythroderma May be due to drugs (Fig. 170) or psoriasis, eczema, pityriasis rubra pilaris and cutaneous T-cell lymphoma.

Management

Withdrawal of offending drug; systemic steroids occasionally; sunblocks when photosensitive component.

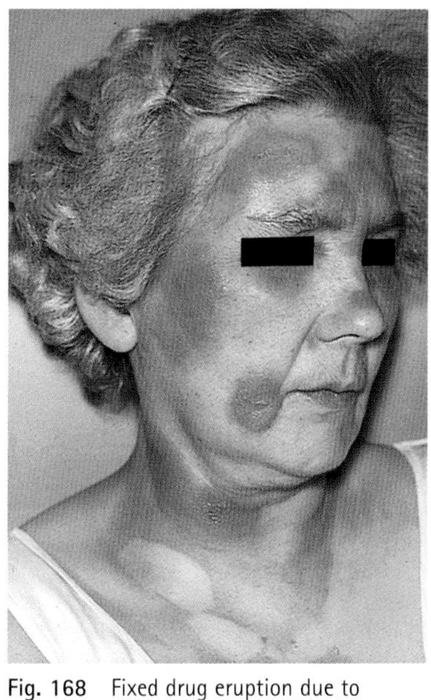

Fig. 168 Fixed drug eruption due to barbiturates, sulphonamides, etc.

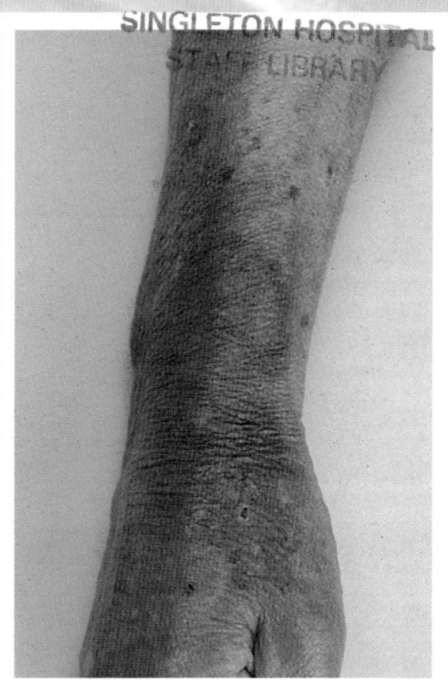

Fig. 169 Amiodarone pigmentation.

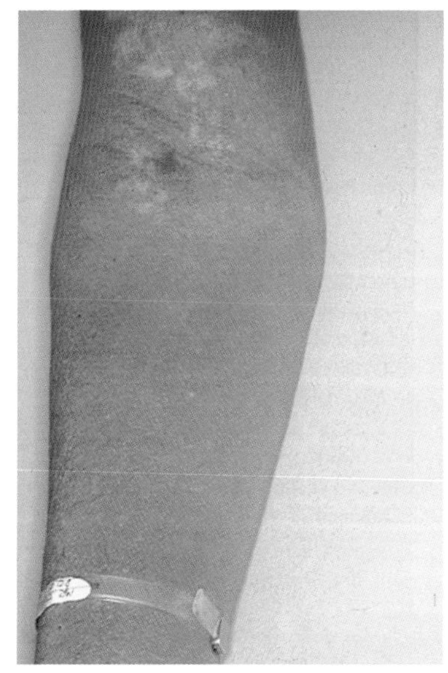

Fig. 170 Drug-induced erythroderma with islands of normal skin.

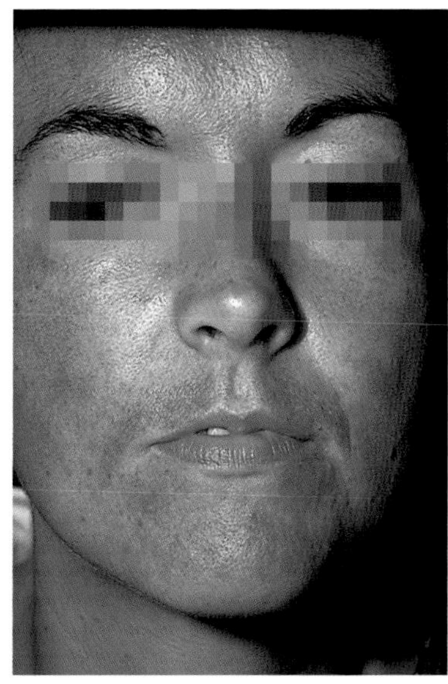

Fig. 171 Melasma.

29 Bacterial infections

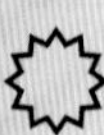

Staphylococcus aureus

Clinical features

Boils, furuncles Staphylococcal hair follicle abscesses—painful, red papules becoming pustular and healing with scarring. Atopy, diabetes and poor hygiene predispose. Patients may carry *S. aureus* in nose, axillae or perineum between attacks.

Folliculitis (Fig. 172) Superficial staphylococcal infection of hair follicles, with small discrete pustules of beard, neck, scalp, buttocks and limbs.

Management

Antibiotics, usually flucloxacillin. Recurrent infections require swabs and appropriate antibiotics. Treat carriers (including family members) with antibiotic nasal cream and antiseptic detergent or powder.

Streptococcus pyogenes

Clinical features

Erysipelas Due to superficial infection with streptococci—tender, red and oedematous skin with a sharply demarcated, indurated edge.

Cellulitis (Figs 173 & 174) A deeper streptococcal infection manifested by lesions with an ill-defined edge. It commonly involves face and legs, and there may be associated lymphangitis, fever or rigors and systemic toxicity. Diabetes, incompetent lymphatics and poor health predispose.

Management

Intravenous penicillin. A penicillinase-resistant antibiotic (e.g. flucloxacillin) may need to be added for combined streptococcal/staphylococcal infections. Erythromycin or cephalosporins can be used for those allergic to penicillin.

Corynebacterium minutissimum

Clinical features

Erythrasma Well-demarcated brownish erythema in axillae, groin and toe webs and under breasts (Fig. 175) with superficial scaling; fluoresces coral-pink under Wood's light.

Management

Fucidin or imidazole cream; oral erythromycin.

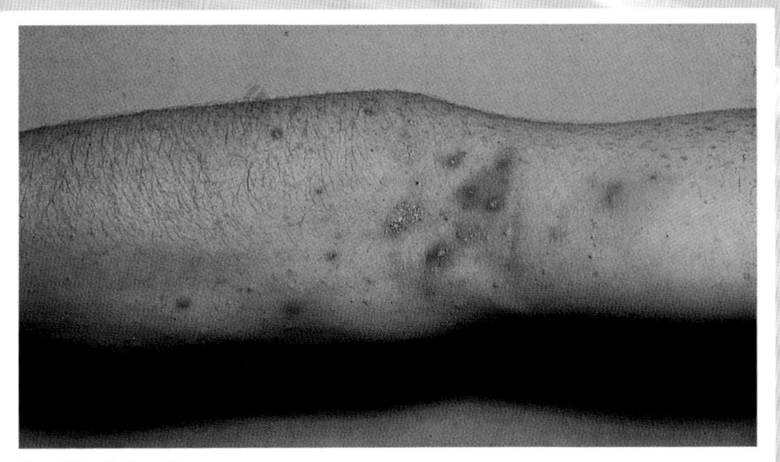

Fig. 172 Folliculitis.

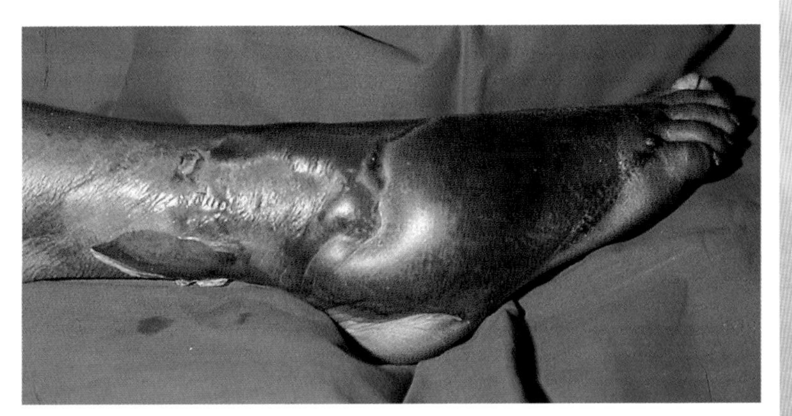

Fig. 173 Bullous cellulitis.

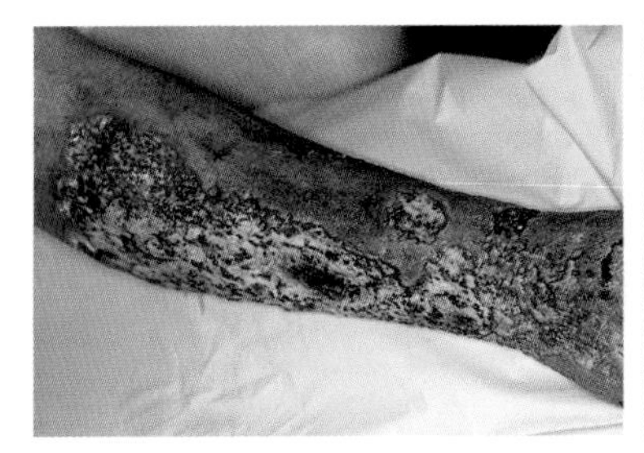

Fig. 174 Extensive ulceration following cellulitis.

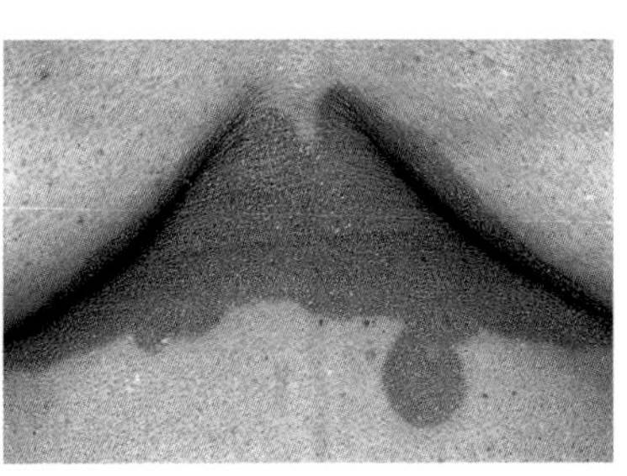

Fig. 175 Erythrasma.

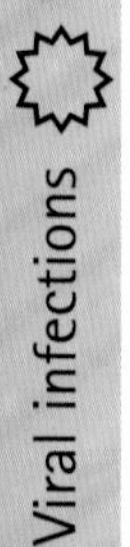

Herpes simplex

Aetiology

Type I virus normally causes herpes labialis, and type II causes genital infections.

Clinical features

Primary herpes simplex (Fig. 176) mainly occurs in children as stomatitis, fever and lymphadenopathy. Recurrent infections are characterized by *herpes labialis* ('cold sore') with small, closely grouped vesicles on an erythematous base. *Eczema herpeticum* occurs in patients with atopic eczema and in the immunosuppressed.

Management

Use topical aciclovir for cold sores or mild localized disease, and oral aciclovir for severe or generalized herpes.

Herpes zoster

Aetiology

Varicella-zoster virus (dormant in dorsal root ganglion after childhood chickenpox).

Clinical features

Pain in the affected dermatome. After 1–3 days, there are clustered, red papules which become vesicular, then pustular (Fig. 177). There may be fever, malaise and lymphadenopathy. Pain may persist for months. Involvement of ophthalmic division of trigeminal nerve may cause keratitis or blindness. Dissemination occurs in the immunosuppressed.

Management

Oral aciclovir for more severe attacks, in older patients and in the immunosuppressed. For post-herpetic neuralgia, use analgesics, carbamazepine, gabapentin, tricyclic antidepressants.

Orf

Aetiology

A para-poxvirus infection acquired from infected lambs.

Clinical features

Firm, dusky or haemorrhagic pustule or bulla, usually on hand (Fig. 178), resolving in 3–6 weeks. Often associated lymphangitis, adenitis and secondary erythema multiforme.

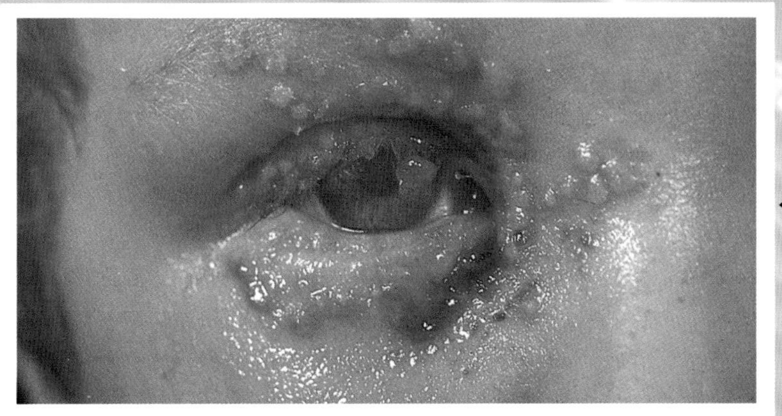

Fig. 176 Herpes simplex. A pustular and crusted eruption with fever, malaise and prostration.

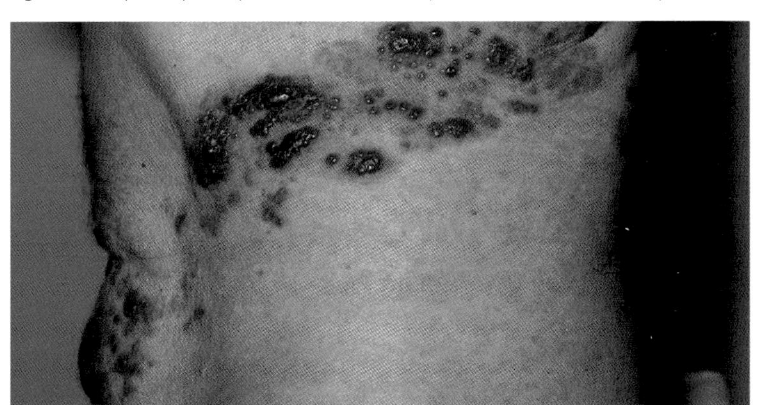

Fig. 177 Typical dermatomal distribution of herpes zoster.

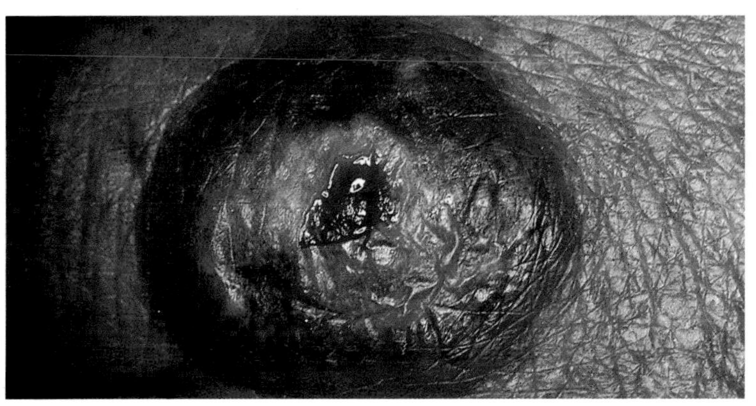

Fig. 178 Orf.

31 HIV/AIDS

Aetiology

HIV-1 and HIV-2 are human T-cell lymphotropic retroviruses that induce progressive, predominantly cell-mediated immunosuppression (AIDS). HIV-2 is geographically very limited, predominantly found in West Africa, and seems less virulent with a slower progression to AIDS. In the absence of antiretroviral treatment, progression to severe immunosuppression may lead to a range of opportunistic infections, several opportunistic neoplasms and direct tissue effects of HIV infection, such as HIV dementia.

Clinical features

It is useful to consider four stages of HIV infection:

1. Acute HIV infection (primary infection or 'seroconversion illness')—approximately 70% experience an infectious mononucleosis-like illness, typically with transient erythematous macular rash on trunk, maculopapular eruptions of upper body or face and papulosquamous eruptions of palms and soles.
2. Clinically latent period: asymptomatic for months or years (average 8–10 years), but high virus and CD4 lymphocyte turnover during this period.
3. 'Pre-AIDS': minor recurrent symptoms, non-specific malaise and, often, persistent general lymphadenopathy associated with low CD4 count, mild neutropenia, hypergammaglobulinaemia. Without antiretroviral treatment, there is risk of progression to the fourth stage.
4. Advanced HIV disease and AIDS:
   - anorexia, diarrhoea, weight loss
   - opportunistic infections, especially fungal (e.g. pneumocystis pneumonia, candida oesophagitis, crytococcal meningitis), bacterial (recurrent pneumococcal pneumonia), mycobacterial (tuberculosis, disseminated *M. avium*), protozoal (e.g. cryptosporidial diarrhoea, toxoplasma encephalitis), viral (e.g. chronic herpes simplex virus infection, cytomegalovirus [CMV] retinitis).

Seborrhoeic dermatitis (Fig. 132, p. 83) This and a papulopruritic eruption (itchy folliculitis) are common during the later symptomatic stages.

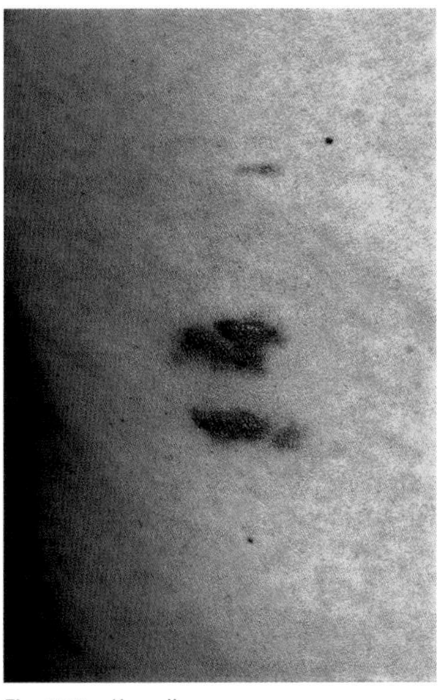

Fig. 179 Kaposi's sarcoma.

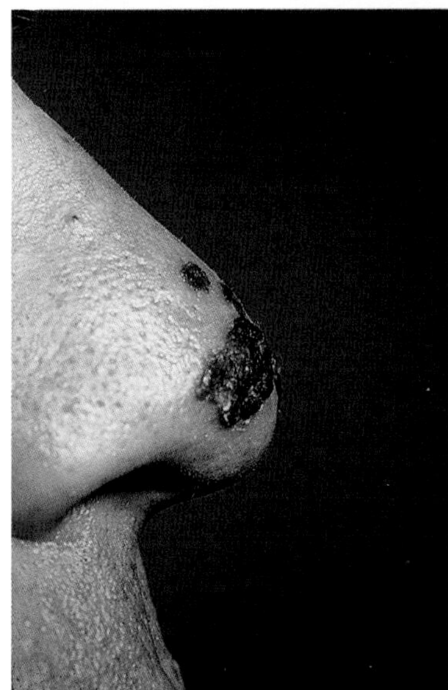

Fig. 181 Herpes simplex.

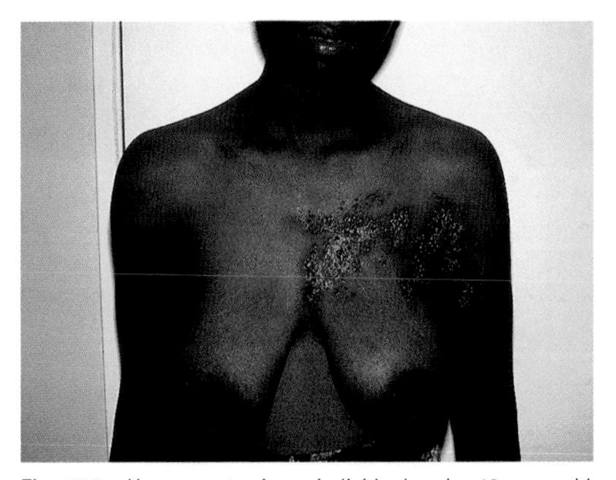

Fig. 180 Herpes zoster in an individual under 40 years old is suggestive of HIV or immunosuppression.

Kaposi's sarcoma A multifocal endothelial cell neoplasm seen predominantly in homosexual men with AIDS (much less frequent since advent of highly active antiretroviral treatment) and also in Africa. Purple or reddish-brown macules, nodules or plaques appear, often in skin creases or on nose or hard palate (Fig. 179, p. 111), caused by infection with human herpes virus (human herpes virus-8, HHV-8; also known as Kaposi's sarcoma associated herpes virus, KSHV), which is transmitted by sexual and other close contact.

Skin infections Herpes zoster (Fig. 180, p. 111), herpes simplex (Fig. 181, p. 111), viral warts, molluscum contagiosum, candidiasis, other fungal infections, including cryptococcus and exotic organisms such as histoplasma, *Penicillium marneffei* (Fig 182), etc., occur secondary to severe immune dysfunction and may be atypical and severe.

Oral hairy leukoplakia (associated with Epstein–Barr virus) Presents as asymptomatic, vertically ribbed keratinized plaques on the lateral borders of the tongue, usually in homosexual men (Fig. 183).

Bacillary angiomatosis
Vascular proliferation caused by disseminated infection with *Bartonella henselae*, the bacterium that causes cat scratch disease in the immunocompetent. Red or violaceous papules and nodules may resemble Kaposi's sarcoma; responds to antibiotic therapy.

Drug eruptions and other side effects Common in patients with HIV, especially advanced HIV infection (e.g. cotrimoxazole rash). Antiretroviral treatment may provoke rash, notably non-nucleoside reverse transcriptase inhibitors (NRTI)—i.e. nevirapine and efavirenz. Long-term antiretroviral treatment, particularly with stavudine, is associated with lipodystrophy (Fig. 184), causing distinctive facial appearance. Zidovudine treatment may be associated with hyperpigmentation.

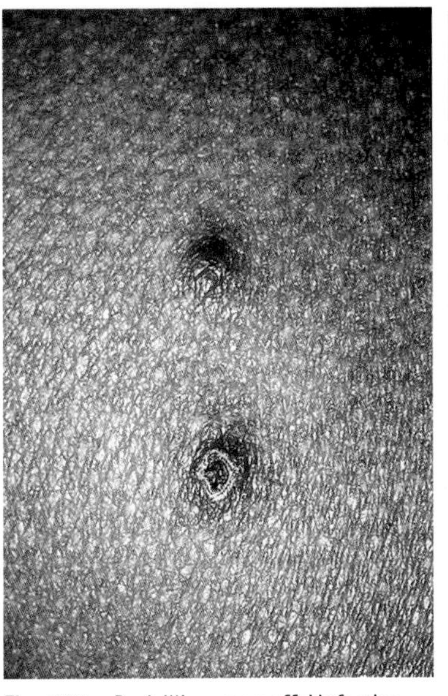

Fig. 182 *Penicillium marneffei* infection.

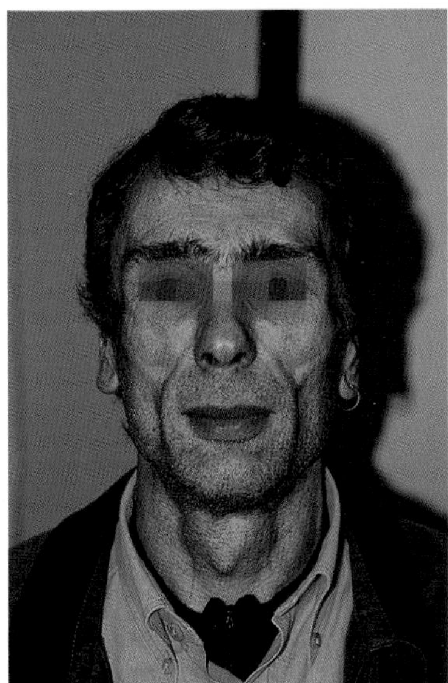

Fig. 184 Lipodystrophy.

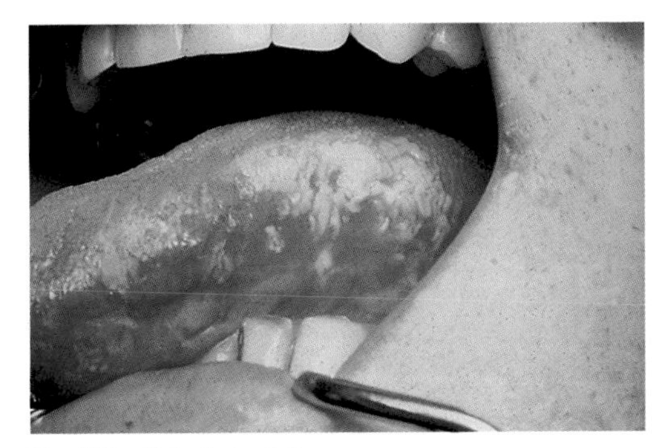

Fig. 183 Hairy leukoplakia.

Other associations Xeroderma, eosinophilic folliculitis (Fig. 185), thrombocytopenic purpura, worsening of psoriasis, widespread granuloma annulare, demodiciosis, prurigo, gingivitis, angular stomatitis, extensive pityriasis versicolor, severe aphthosis (Fig. 186), worsening of eczema, vasculitis, Norwegian scabies and the development of long eyelashes.

Management

Highly active antiretroviral treatment (HAART) has transformed the short- and medium-term prognosis of individuals with HIV infection. Numerous antiretroviral agents are licensed for treatment, and others are in development. Treatment is recommended before the CD4 lymphocyte count falls below 200/mm^3; response to therapy is monitored by measurement of HIV viral load (quantitative test for HIV RNA in blood). A minimum of three drugs is used to minimize risk of development of viral resistance. Selection of antiretroviral drug after treatment failures, and increasingly before starting treatment, may be guided by *in vitro* resistance testing.

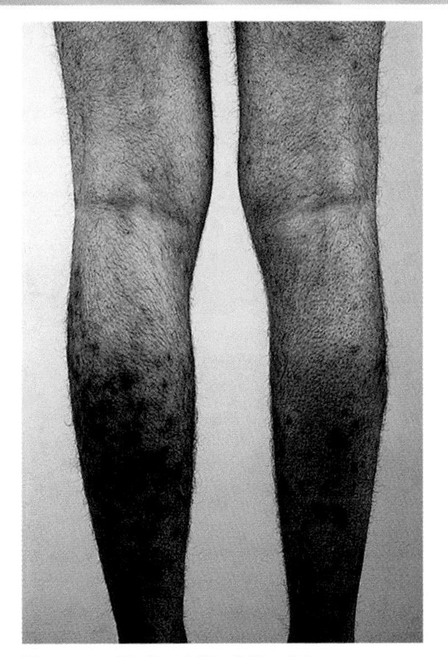

Fig. 185 Eosinophilic folliculitis.

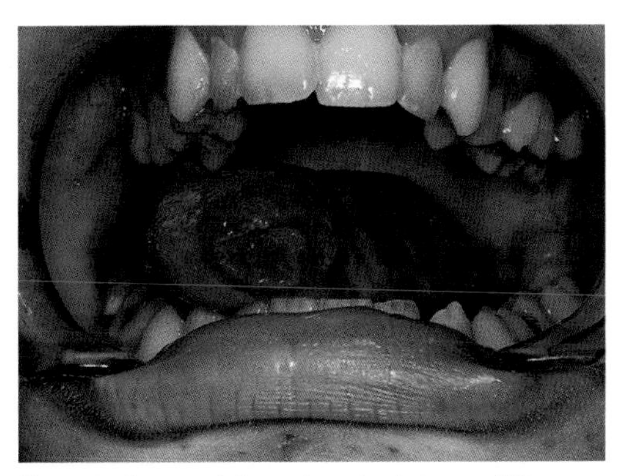

Fig. 186 Severe aphthous ulceration in haemophiliac patient with AIDS.

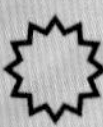

Tineas

Aetiology

Ringworm (tinea) infections. Obtain scrapings for microscopy and culture before beginning treatment. Infections are classified as follows:

- Tinea pedis (athlete's foot) is due to *Trichophyton rubrum*, *T. interdigitale* and *Epidermophyton floccosum*. It is precipitated by hot and humid weather, communal showering, use of swimming pools and occlusive footwear.
- Tinea manuum is predominantly due to *T. rubrum*.
- Tinea cruris is caused by the same organisms as tinea pedis.
- Tinea corporis is caused by all types of ringworm.

Clinical features

Tinea pedis (Figs 187 & 188) Scaling, fissuring or irritation, especially between 4th and 5th toes.

It may be caused not only by dermatophytes but also by candida, other bacteria or maceration. It may be associated with erythema, scaling and occasionally vesicles or pustules on sole of foot.

Tinea manuum (Fig. 189) Characteristically unilateral with scaling of the palm. Exaggerated skin markings are also seen.

Tinea cruris Occurs predominantly in young men. There is well-demarcated erythema and scaling in the groin with central clearing and an 'active' edge (Fig. 190, p. 119).

Tinea corporis Discoid, scaly areas that spread slowly with central clearing. The edge of the lesion may be vesicular (Fig. 191, p. 119).

Management

Topical antifungal agents (e.g. Whitfield's ointment or imidazole or terbinafine creams) for interdigital maceration, lotions for hairy areas. Oral terbinafine, itraconazole or griseofulvin for 2–6 weeks for more severe, recurrent or extensive disease and for palms, soles and hairy areas.

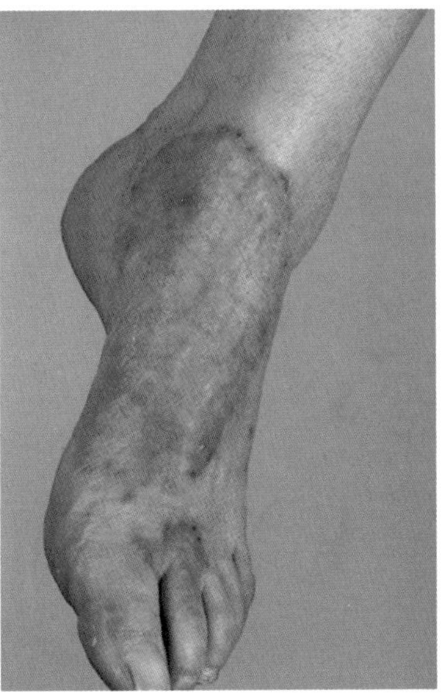

Fig. 187 Tinea pedis.

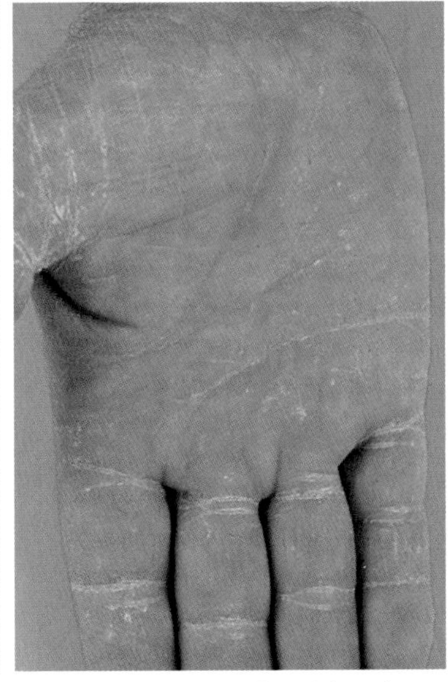

Fig. 189 Unilateral scaling of the palm (tinea manuum).

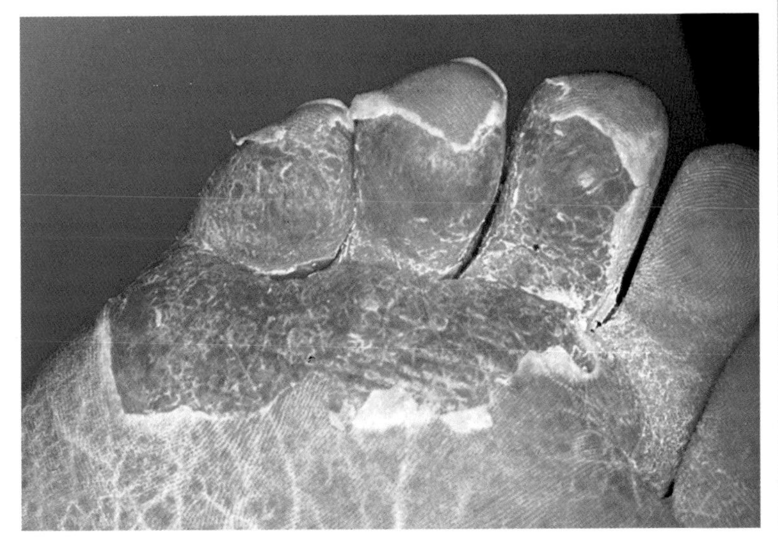

Fig. 188 Dermatophyte infection spreading out from the toes.

Tinea incognito

Aetiology

Ringworm infection modified by topical (or systemic) steroids (Fig. 187, p. 117, and Fig. 192).

Clinical features

The inflammatory response is suppressed by use of steroids. Itching and inflammation are reduced, the margins less distinct and scaling less apparent, yet the lesion is slowly enlarging.

Management

Topical imidazole or terbinafine and systemic antifungal agent (e.g. terbinafine or itraconazole). There may be some rebound increase in inflammation on stopping the steroid.

Majocchi's ringworm granuloma

Aetiology

A foreign body granulomatous reaction due to folliculitis from *Trichophyton* infection (Fig. 192).

Clinical features

Predominantly in adults; an erythematous, scaly plaque on a limb studded with follicular pustules. The plaque is unilateral, but may spread.

Management

Oral systemic antifungal.

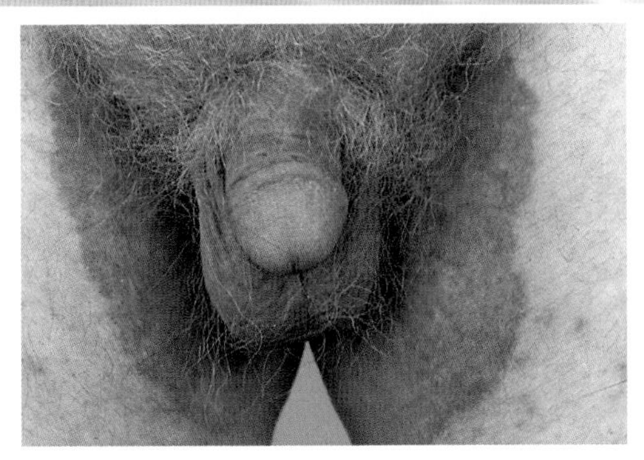

Fig. 190 Tinea cruris.

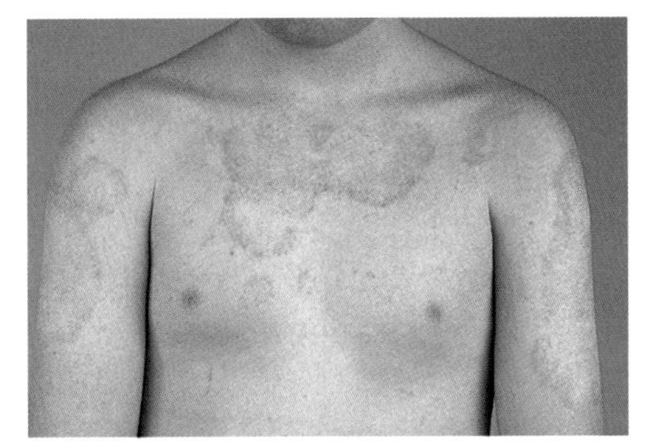

Fig. 191 Tinea corporis.

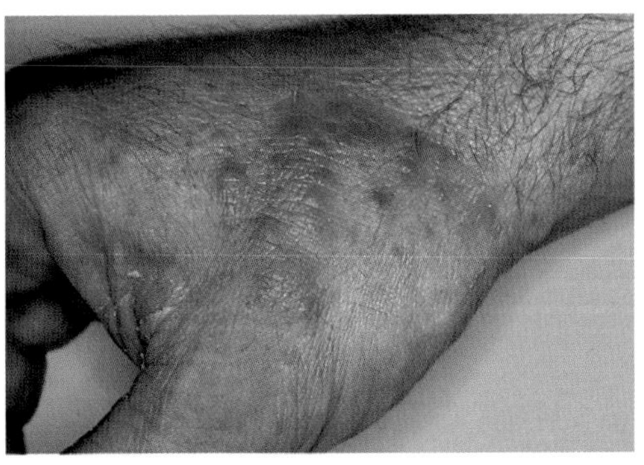

Fig. 192 Majocchi's granuloma.

Pityriasis versicolor (tinea versicolor)

Aetiology

Pityrosporum orbiculare.

Clinical features

The condition is common in hot, humid environments. It presents as hyperpigmented or hypopigmented macules with fine superficial scales (Fig. 193), mostly on the trunk or upper limbs and often more conspicuous following sunbathing. It tends to relapse.

Management

Selenium sulphide or ketoconazole as 'body shampoos' or topical imidazole creams. Oral itraconazole may be used in resistant cases. It may take several months for normal skin colour to return. Intermittent prophylactic treatment may be needed.

Candidiasis

Aetiology

Candida albicans; moisture, warmth, occlusion, antibiotics, steroid treatment, pregnancy, diabetes and immunosuppression all predispose.

Clinical features

Erythema with scaling (Fig. 194) and papular or pustular satellite lesions at and beyond a well-defined irregular edge, affecting skin folds, especially in obese patients (intertrigo). It may be itchy or sore. (See also Napkin candidiasis, p. 10.)

Management

Nystatin or imidazole creams. Eradication of gut and vaginal yeast carriage and oral fluconazole or itraconazole in resistant cases.

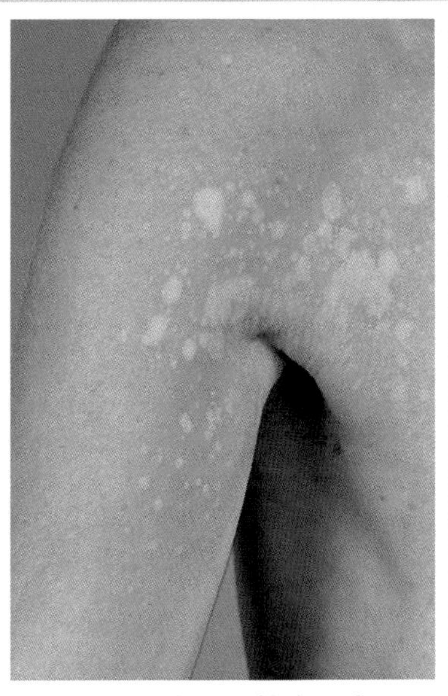

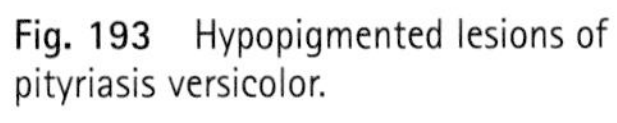

Fig. 193 Hypopigmented lesions of pityriasis versicolor.

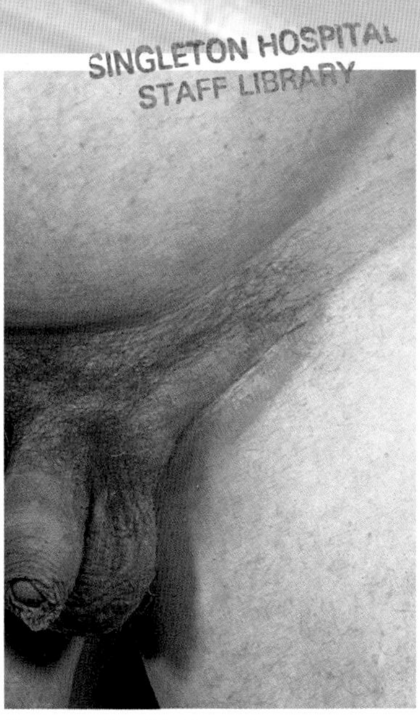

Fig. 194 Candidal intertrigo.

33 Infestations

Scabies

Aetiology

Sarcoptes scabiei var. *hominis*. Eggs are laid in epidermal burrows by the female acarus (mite). Overcrowding and sexual promiscuity predispose.

Clinical features

Pruritus is severe, intractable and worse at night, commencing about 2 weeks after the primary infection when the patient has developed hypersensitivity to the mite. Characteristic burrows (Fig. 195) are seen in finger webs and on flexor aspects of wrists, palms and feet, with characteristic papules on penis (Fig. 196), on buttocks and around areolae. Vesicles may occur, but excoriations are more common (Fig. 197). Impetigo may coexist. Indurated, inflammatory nodules are sometimes seen on the scrotum and elsewhere. Lesions do not affect the head, except in infants, who often also have lesions around the umbilicus. The acarus can be demonstrated by scraping a burrow and examining the contents in 20% KOH under a microscope.

Management

Topical malathion 0.5%, permethrin 1% or benzyl benzoate application b.p., applied at night from neck to soles and repeated if necessary 1 week later. Children are probably best treated with aqueous malathion lotion. Crotamiton cream or lotion can be used later to treat pruritus or to prevent recurrence. Treatment should be combined with a change of contact clothing and bedding. All close contacts and all members of the household must be treated whether clinically affected or not. (NB: care is needed in the choice of treatment in children <6 months old and pregnant women.) Treatment may need to include the head in young children, the elderly or immunocompromised and in cases of treatment failure.

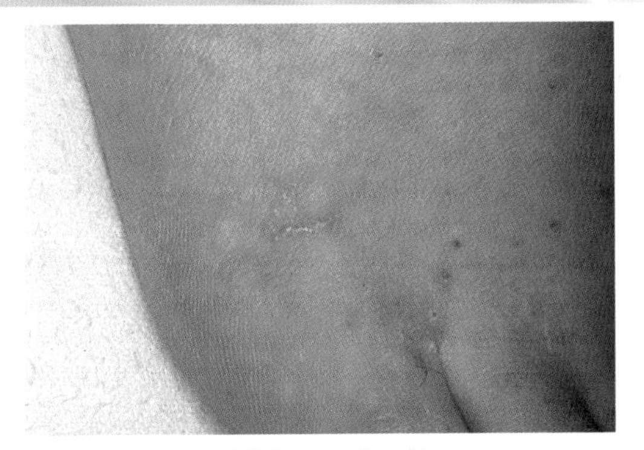

Fig. 195 Characteristic burrow of scabies.

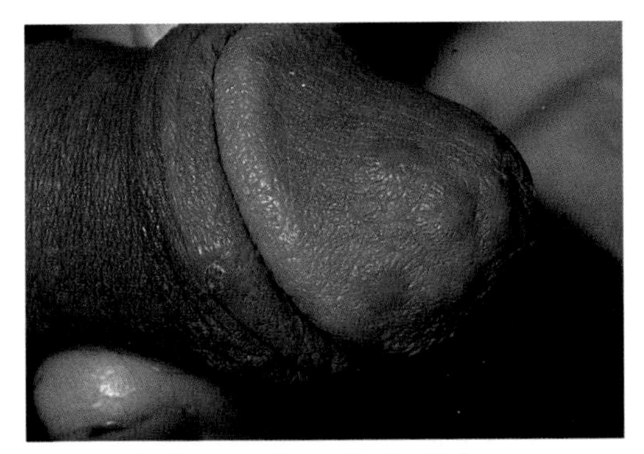

Fig. 196 Persistent penile papules (scabies).

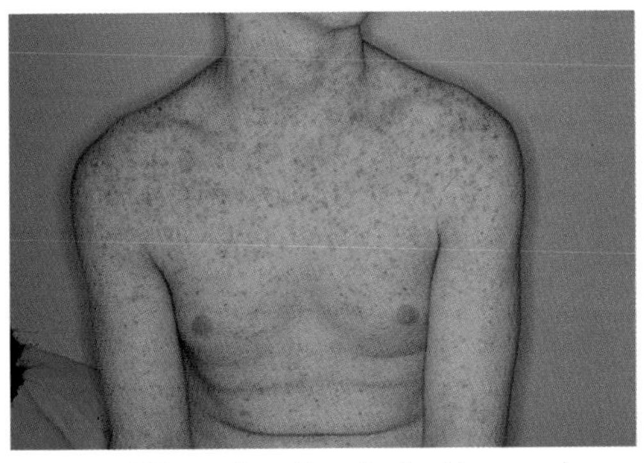

Fig. 197 Widespread pruritic rash of scabies.

Lice

Aetiology

Lice are translucent, wingless insects. Poor hygiene and crowded conditions predispose.

Clinical features

Head louse See page 26.

Body louse Asymptomatic pinpoint red macules. Pruritus, excoriations, papular urticaria and secondary infection, with hyperpigmentation in chronic cases (Fig. 198). Lice and eggs are found in the seams of clothing.

Pubic louse Often transmitted by sexual contact. There is intense pruritus of the pubic region. The eggs (nits) appear as grains of sand attached to the hair shafts.

Management

Remove nits with a fine-toothed metal comb. Treat with 0.5% carbaryl, 0.5% phenothrin or 1% permethrin or 0.5% malathion lotion. Contacts must also be treated. A thorough disinfection of clothing is necessary.

Larva migrans

Aetiology

The larvae of various worms (e.g. *Ancylostoma braziliense, Strongyloides stercoralis).*

Clinical features

The larvae penetrate the skin of feet, hands or buttocks. They migrate, producing intensely itchy, raised, red serpentine lines (Fig. 199).

Management

Local application of 10% thiabendazole suspension or oral albendazole or ivermectin.

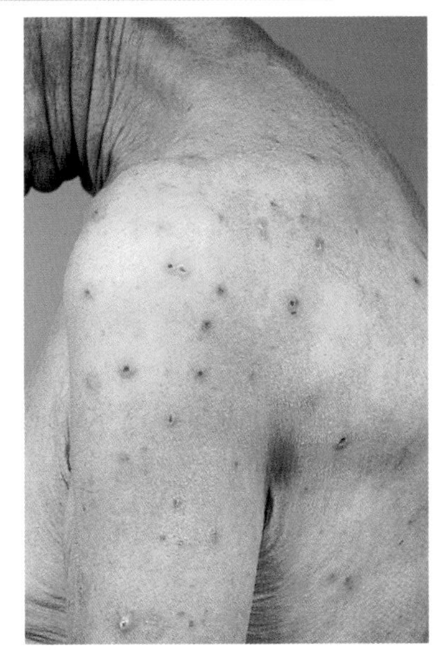

Fig. 198 Generalized excoriations (pediculosis corporis).

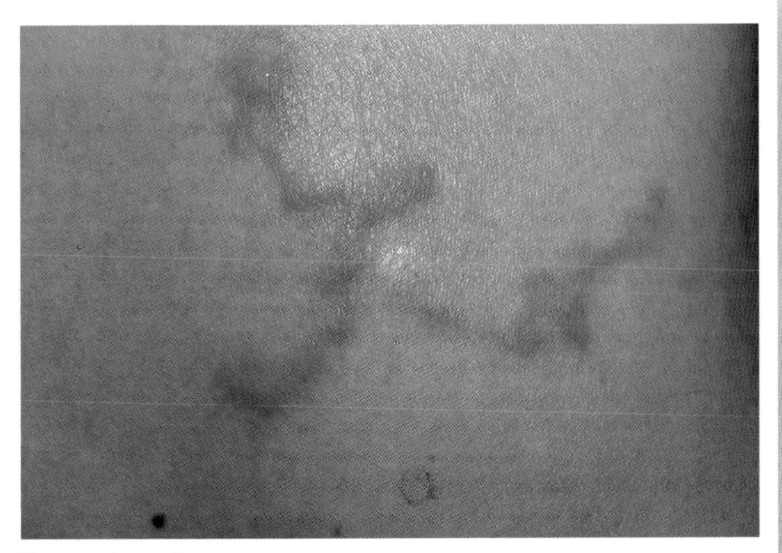

Fig. 199 Larva migrans.

34 Adult benign tumours

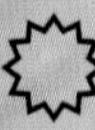

	Seborrhoeic wart (basal cell papilloma)
Aetiology	Often familial.
Clinical features	Common in both sexes in middle to later life, usually on the trunk, increasing in number and size with age. Characteristically yellow-brown or black and greasy, with a rough craggy surface (Fig. 200).
Differential diagnosis	Malignant melanoma; pigmented basal cell carcinoma.
Management	Curettage (with application of superficial styptic); cryotherapy. Histology if solitary or in doubt.

	Skin tags (fibroepithelial polyps)
Aetiology	Familial: obesity, pregnancy.
Clinical features	Multiple, soft, round and peduncular with a narrow base (Fig. 201). These characteristically occur on the neck, axillae and groin; often coexisting with seborrhoeic warts.
Management	'Snip' and cautery; diathermy.

	Solar lentigos ('senile'/actinic lentigos)
Aetiology	Excessive exposure to sunlight.
Clinical features	Light brown macules, often multiple, occurring on light-exposed skin of fair-skinned individuals (Fig. 202).
Differential diagnosis	Lentigo maligna.
Management	None. Cryotherapy, sunscreens, ruby laser. Biopsy and histology if in doubt.

	Campbell de Morgan spots (cherry angiomas; haemangiomas)
Clinical features	Multiple, small bright red spots (Fig. 203), often familial, on trunk of middle-aged and elderly.
Management	None; diathermy, vascular laser.

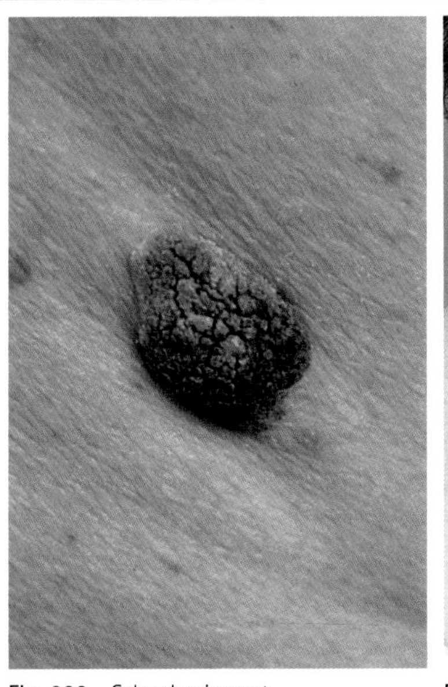

Fig. 200 Seborrhoeic wart.

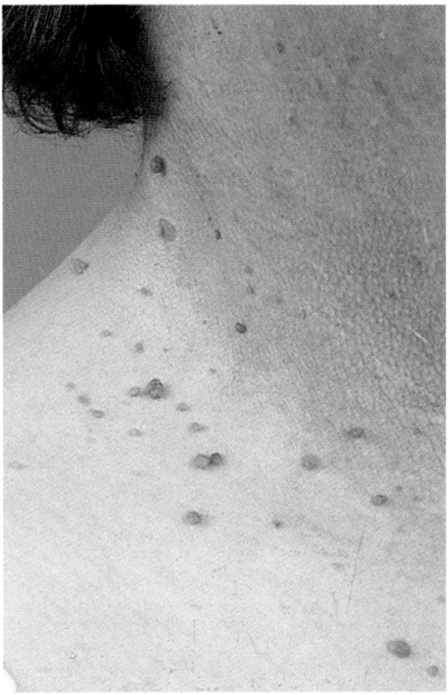

Fig. 201 Skin tags.

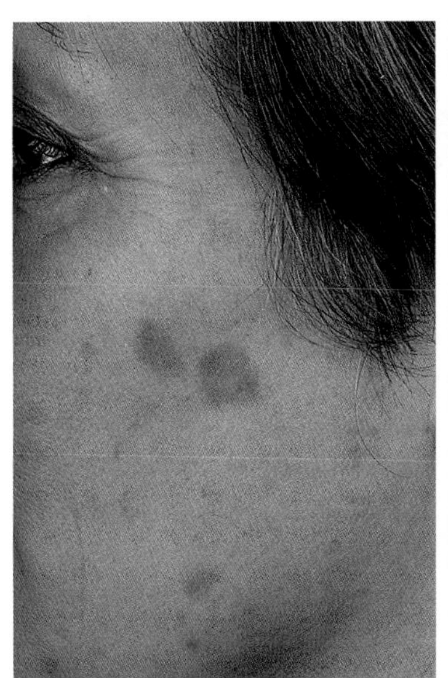

Fig. 202 Solar lentigos.

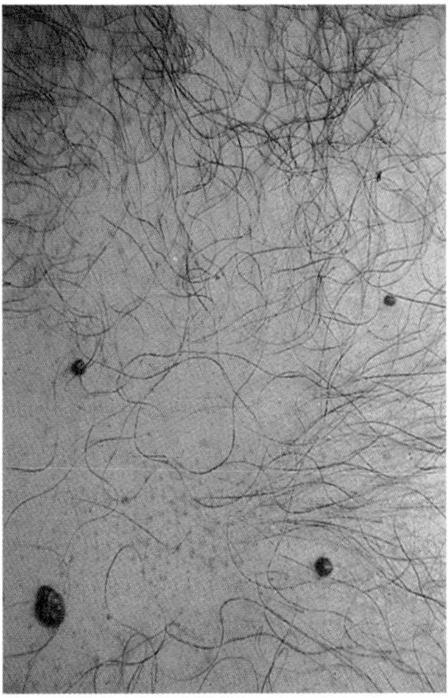

Fig. 203 Campbell de Morgan angiomas.

35 Premalignant tumours

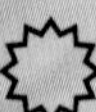

Solar keratoses (actinic keratoses)

Aetiology Chronic exposure to UVL.

Clinical features Commoner in the fair-skinned or ex-patriots living in sunnier climates, in middle to old age. Affect the backs of hands, forehead, scalp, temples, nose, cheeks and ears, with rough, adherent crusts on an erythematous base (Fig. 204).

Management Curettage and trichloracetic acid; cryotherapy; photodynamic therapy, 5-fluorouracil, 3% diclofenac or imiquimod creams for multiple lesions.

Bowen's disease/Leukoplakia/Erythroplasia

Aetiology Previous exposure to UVL, arsenic or other carcinogen; pre-invasive intraepidermal carcinoma.

Clinical features Appearing anywhere on the skin (Figs 205 & 206) as asymptomatic, erythematous, well-demarcated, scaly patches or as 'velvet' or white patches on mucosal surfaces. Ulceration suggests invasive growth.

Management Surgical excision; cryotherapy; photodynamic therapy, 5-fluorouracil cream.

Keratoacanthoma

Clinical features Occurs in middle to old age, mainly on sun-exposed skin of face or dorsum of hands. A flesh-coloured papule enlarges rapidly over 8–10 weeks with a central keratin-filled crater (Fig. 207). Spontaneous involution leaves depressed scar.

Management Surgical excision, shave or curettage and cautery, or biopsy followed by superficial radiotherapy or intralesional methotrexate.

Oral leukoplakia

See page 134.

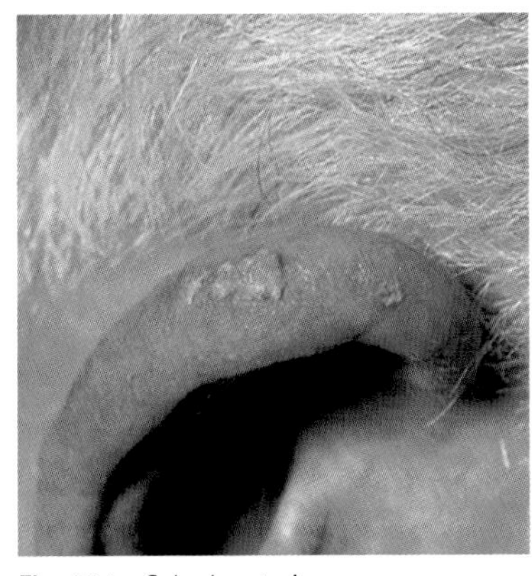

Fig. 204 Solar keratosis.

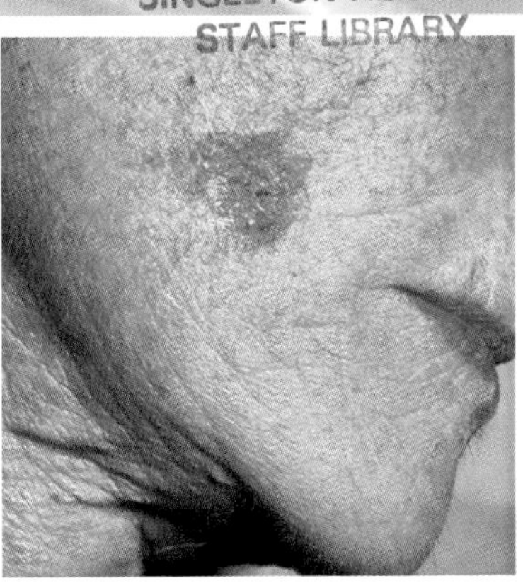

Fig. 205 Localized patch of Bowen's disease on the face.

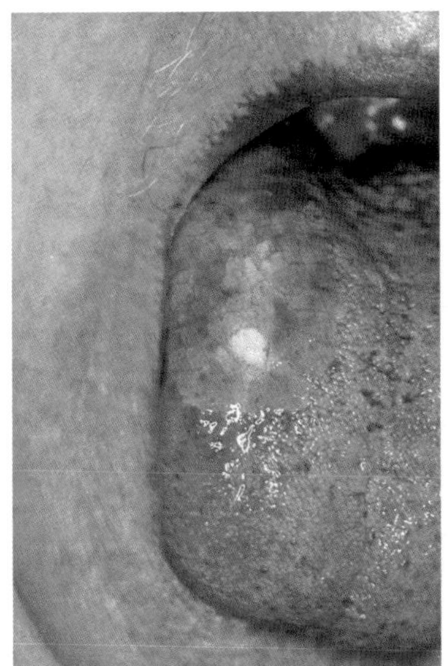

Fig. 206 Leukoplakia (carcinoma in situ). Well-demarcated white patches on tongue.

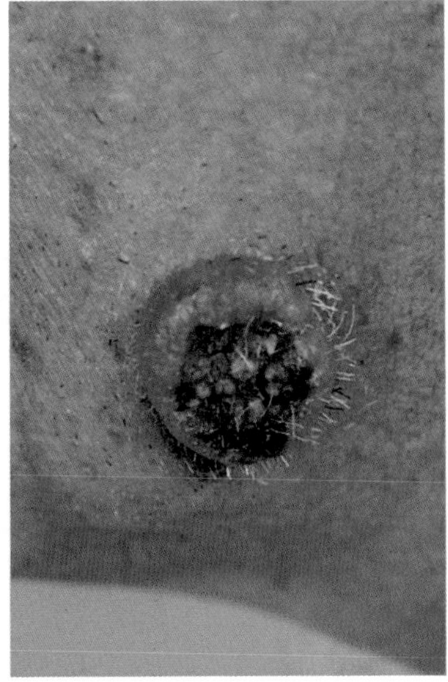

Fig. 207 Typical keratoacanthoma.

36 Tumours

Basal cell carcinoma (BCC)

Aetiology

Chronic cutaneous sun-damage or exposure to arsenicals or radiotherapy.

Clinical features

Commonest cutaneous malignancy. It occurs in middle to old age, usually on the head and neck. The lesion classically begins as a raised, pearly or translucent papule with telangiectasia, central ulceration and a typical rolled edge (Fig. 208). It may be pigmented, multifocal (Fig. 209) or sclerotic/morphoeic. Fibrosing or penetrating BCC may erode underlying tissues.

Management

Surgical excision; radiotherapy; curettage and cautery. Superficial multifocal BCCs are sometimes treated with aggressive cryotherapy or photodynamic therapy.

Squamous cell carcinomas (SCC)

Aetiology

Exposure to sunlight. Industrial carcinogens and long-standing ulcers also predispose.

Clinical features

May develop 'de novo' or on previously sun-damaged skin or on a background of solar keratosis, Bowen's disease or leukoplakia. The lesions begin as nodules on a firm indurated base, ulcerating as they enlarge (Fig. 210), commonly on the backs of hands and face, especially the lower lip and ear. Metastases are uncommon in the sun-induced type, but more frequent in 'de novo' SCC or on a background of Bowen's disease or leukoplakia (Figs 205 & 206, p. 129).

Management

Surgical excision.

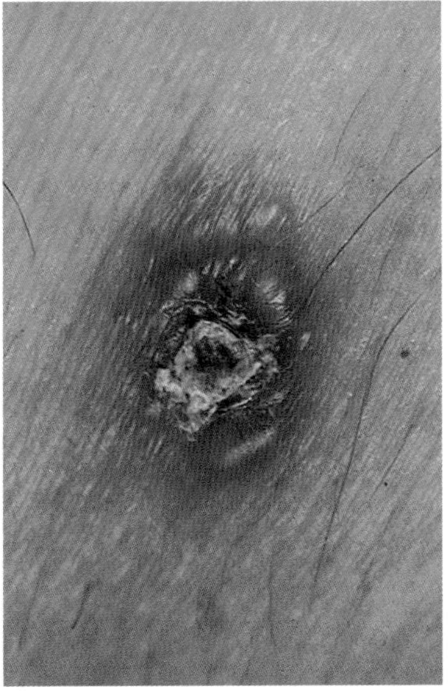

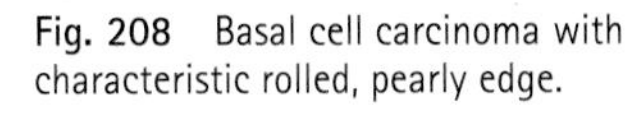

Fig. 208 Basal cell carcinoma with characteristic rolled, pearly edge.

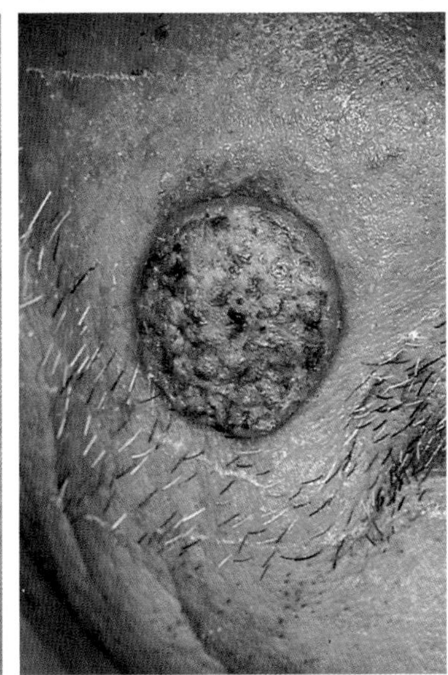

Fig. 210 Squamous cell carcinoma of the face.

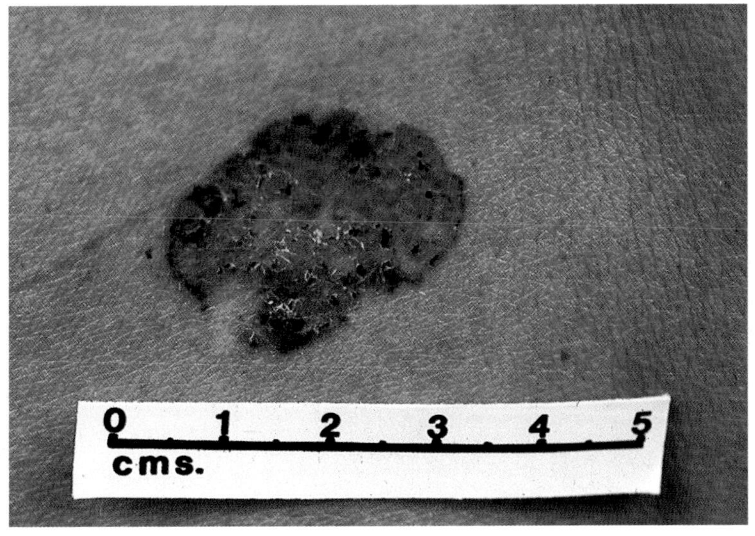

Fig. 209 Superficial multifocal pigmented BCC.

Lentigo maligna

Aetiology

Intraepidermal, pre-invasive, malignant melanoma.

Clinical features

Appears in middle to old age as a flat brown stain with an irregular, well-demarcated edge, slowly enlarging with variable pigmentation. It most commonly affects the face. Nodular malignant melanoma may develop after many years (Fig. 211).

Management

Aggressive cryotherapy or superficial radiotherapy in the macular phase. Excision if small or nodular.

Malignant melanoma

Aetiology

Excessive exposure to sunlight.

Clinical features

Any 'new' pigmented mole or one that changes its character in adult life should be regarded as malignant melanoma until proved otherwise. Rapidly becoming one of the commoner forms of cancer in those between the ages of 20 and 50 years. Prognosis worsens rapidly, and early referral is obligatory. Superficial spreading melanoma starts as a slightly elevated, irregular brown or black patch (Fig. 212). Nodule formation indicates a vertically invasive stage (Figs 213 & 214). Nodular melanoma has a poorer prognosis. Melanoma under the nail may be mistaken for subungual haemorrhage.

Management

Early wide excision with block dissection of lymph nodes if involved.

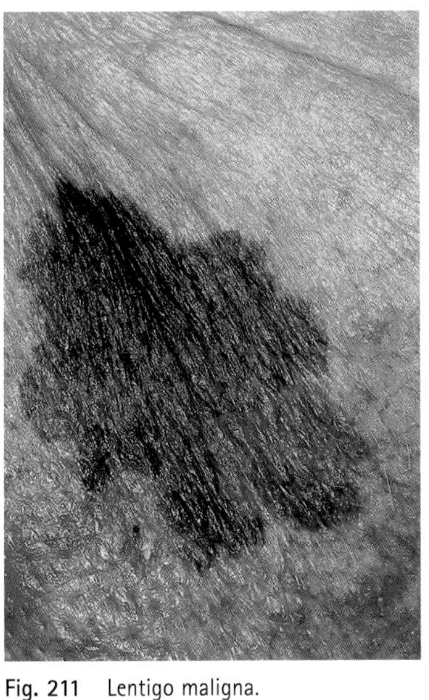

Fig. 211 Lentigo maligna.

Fig. 212 Superficial spreading melanoma.

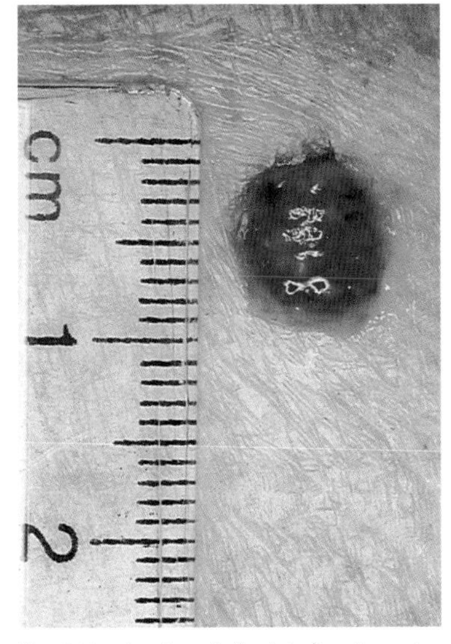

Fig. 213 Amelanotic (nodular) malignant melanoma.

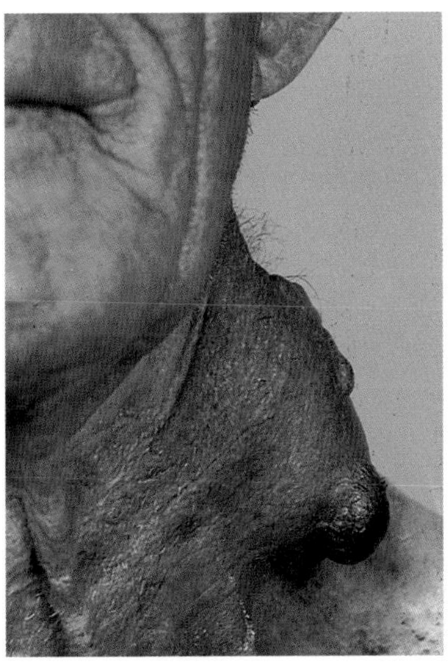

Fig. 214 Nodular malignant melanoma with lymphadenopathy.

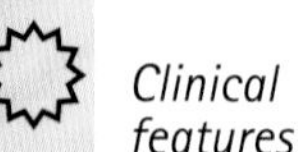

37 Oral conditions

Lichen planus

Clinical features — Mucous membrane lesions (Fig. 215) occur in 50% of cases but may occur in isolation. Candidiasis, secondary syphilis, leukoplakia and lichenoid reaction to dental amalgam must be differentiated.

Management — Symptomatic.

Geographic tongue

Clinical features — Benign, inflammatory disorder of unknown cause, usually asymptomatic. Multiple smooth, erythematous patches migrate in a map-like pattern on the dorsum of the tongue.

Recurrent aphthae

Clinical features — Common disorder of buccal mucosae, tongue and gingival folds. Small, erythematous pustules rapidly break down to form painful shallow ulcers (Fig. 216) that heal in 7–10 days.

Management — Symptomatic; tetracycline mouthwash; topical steroids. Exclude haematinic deficiencies and coeliac disease.

Black hairy tongue

Clinical features — May follow treatment with antibiotics and cytotoxics. The elongated papillae may be yellow-brown or black.

Leukoplakia

Clinical features — Small, discrete, white patches or more extensive, leathery plaques on an atrophic erythematous base (Fig. 206, p. 129). Tobacco smoking and recurrent trauma predispose. Risk of malignant change.

Management — Excision or biopsy, cryotherapy.

Pemphigus

Clinical features — Mucosal or gingival erosions (Fig. 217) are a common presenting feature (see p. 98). Differentiate from Stevens–Johnson syndrome (Figs 106 & 166, pp. 67 & 103).

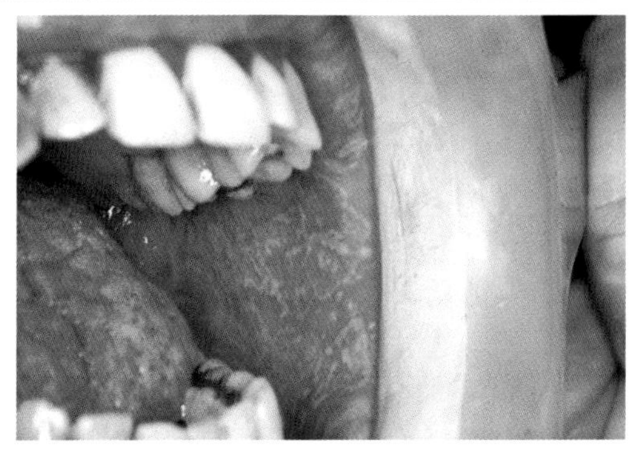

Fig. 215 Bluish-white lace-like striae of oral lichen planus.

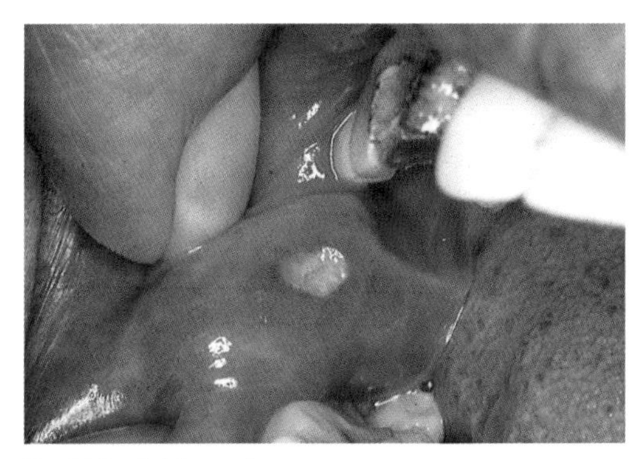

Fig. 216 Aphthous ulcer.

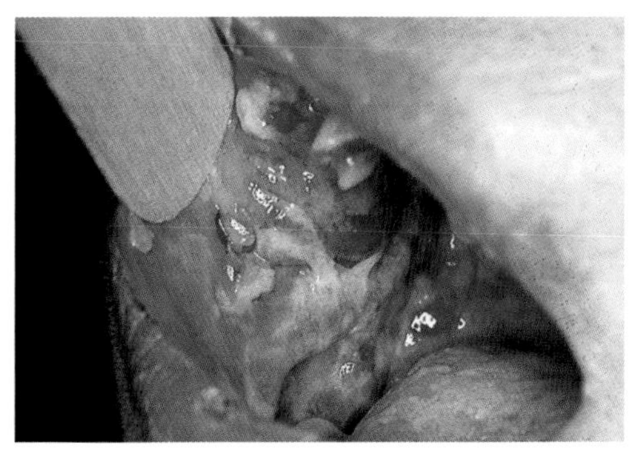

Fig. 217 Mucosal pemphigus.

38 Genitals

Lichen planus

Clinical features

Characteristic violaceous papules with fine lacework of white striae occur on the penile shaft, glans and prepuce (Fig. 218) or on the inner surface of labia. Annular and erosive forms may also occur.

Management

Topical steroids if symptomatic (see also p. 94).

Lichen sclerosus

Clinical features

Uncommon autoimmune disease mainly affecting women. Ivory-white or violaceous areas occur on the perianal and vulval regions with 'cigarette paper' atrophy. There may be follicular plugging, erosions and fissuring, sclerosis and purpura (Fig. 219). In men, the glans penis and foreskin may be involved, leading to phimosis or meatal stricture. Dyspareunia, soreness and pruritus often cause distress. The condition is potentially premalignant (more often in women).

Management

Potent topical steroids initially and for phimosis or meatal strictures. Surgery may be necessary.

Psoriasis

Clinical features

Well-defined smooth, erythematous plaques on genitalia (Fig. 220). Important to differentiate from erythroplasia of Queyrat (Bowen's disease) (see also p. 128).

Management

Mild to moderate strength steroid creams.

Plasma cell balanitis

Clinical features

A well-localized, shiny and exudative balanitis, often non-specific in nature, with prominent plasma cells on histology (Fig. 221). Occurs especially in the uncircumcised. Exclude erythroplasia and specific infections.

Management

Frequent wet soaks, steroid/antibacterial creams and antibiotics if indicated. In resistant cases, circumcision is indicated.

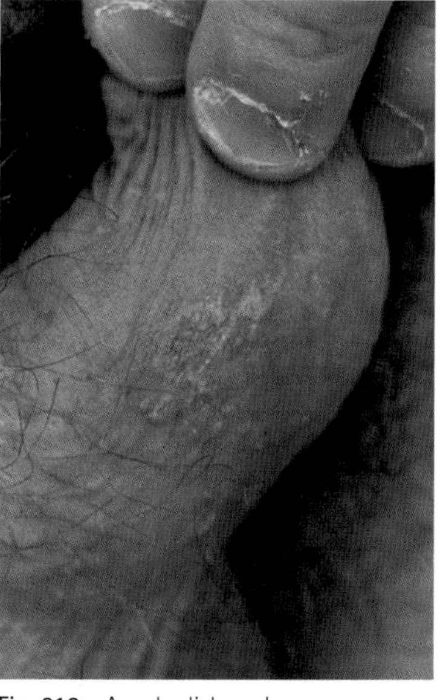
Fig. 218 Annular lichen planus.

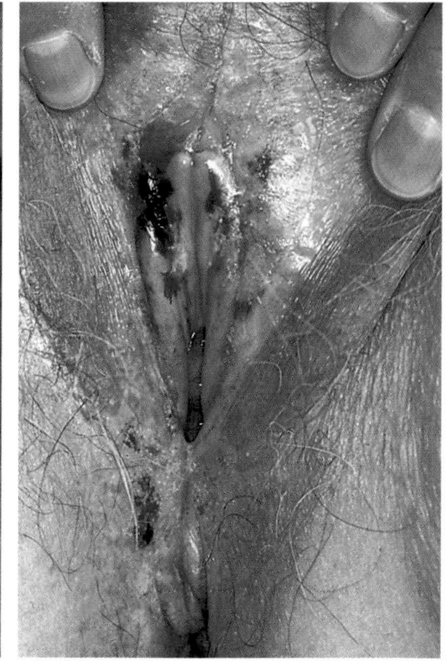
Fig. 219 Lichen sclerosus of perineum.

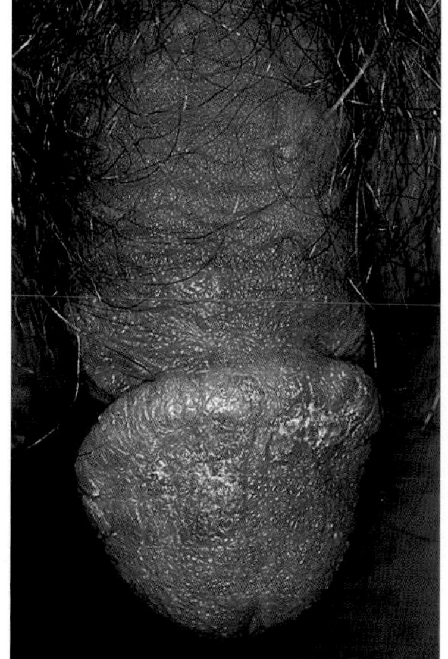
Fig. 220 Psoriasis/Reiter's syndrome with involvement of glans penis.

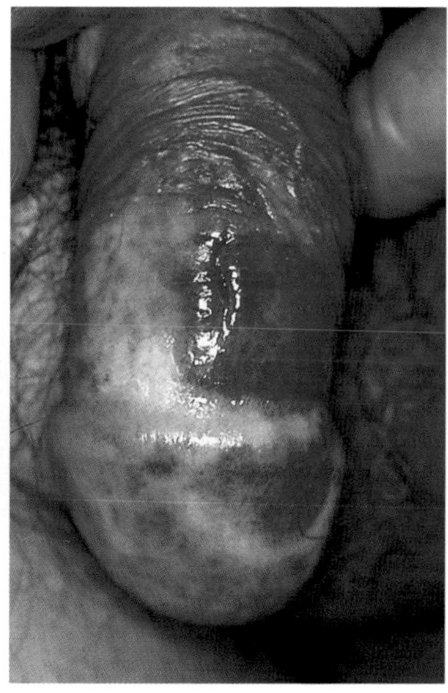
Fig. 221 Non-specific or plasma cell balanitis.

39 Nails

Onychogryphosis

Aetiology
Age, trauma and ill-fitting shoes predispose.

Clinical features
Usually affects the great toenails. Hypertrophy progresses to typical 'ram's horn' (Fig. 222).

Management
Regular chiropody.

Onycholysis

Aetiology
Causes include trauma (both physical and chemical), infection, psoriasis, eczema, poor circulation, photosensitivity to certain drugs (e.g. tetracyclines), and thyroid disease (Fig. 223).

Clinical features
Lifting of the nail plate distally. A secondary pseudomonas infection may develop.

Management
Reduce trauma. Keep nails short and dry.

Onychomycosis

Aetiology
Usually *Trichophyton rubrum* or *T. mentagraphytes.*

Clinical features
White or yellowish discolouration. The nail becomes thickened with subungual hyperkeratosis, splinter haemorrhages and onycholysis (Fig. 224).

Management
Terbinafine for 3 months, or itraconazole, 1 week a month for 3 months.

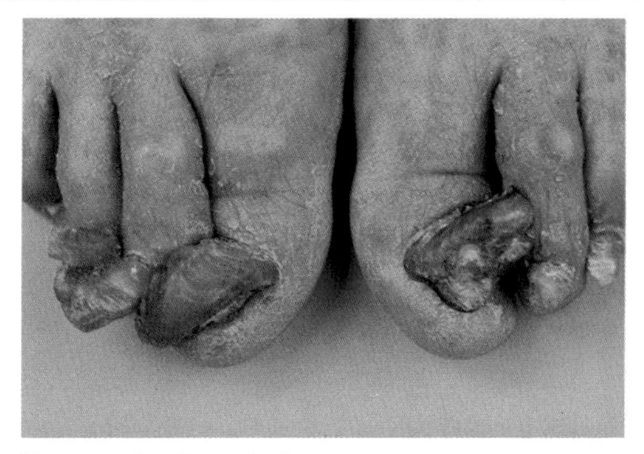

Fig. 222 Onychogryphosis.

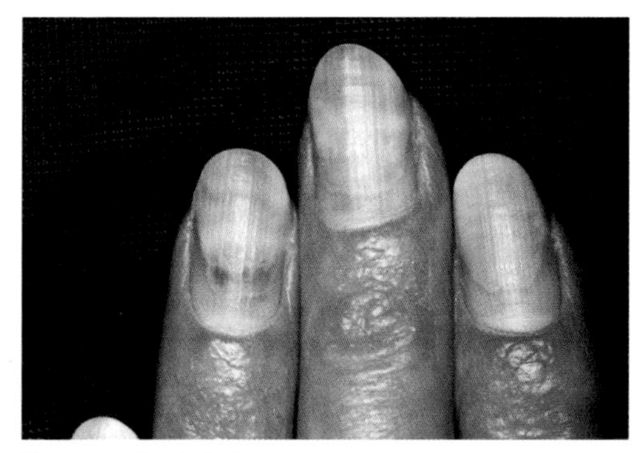

Fig. 223 Onycholysis.

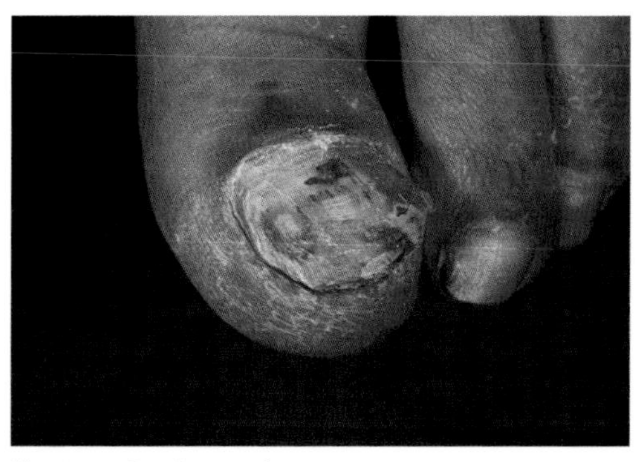

Fig. 224 Onychomycosis.

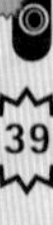
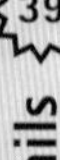
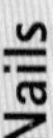
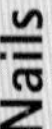
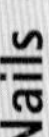
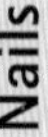
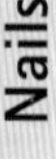
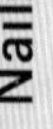
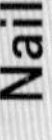
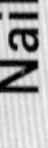

Psoriasis

Clinical features

The nails may be involved in the absence of psoriasis elsewhere with pitting, onycholysis (Fig. 225), subungual hyperkeratosis, yellowing and thickening and splinter haemorrhages.

Management

Generally unrewarding.

Lichen planus

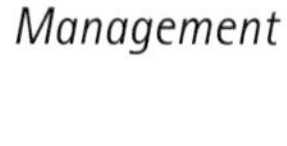

Clinical features

Nail changes can occur in the absence of lesions elsewhere. This may progress to atrophy with scarring (Fig. 226) or even permanent destruction. The cuticle may grow over the base of the nail and attach to the nail plate (pterygium) with increased longitudinal striations of nail plate, ridging and splitting. The nail plate becomes thinned.

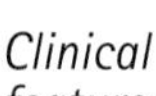
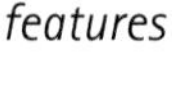
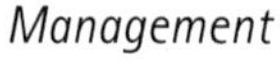

Management

Rarely, intralesional or systemic steroids.

Alopecia areata/Twenty-nail dystrophy

Clinical features

The nail plate becomes dull and roughened, with small, fine, regular pitting (ground glass appearance) (Fig. 227).

Management

No specific treatment.

Eczema/Chronic paronychia

Clinical features

Nail changes can occur in any type of eczema, but are more often seen in atopic eczema. Several changes occur, including transverse irregular ridging and shedding. Onycholysis and chronic paronychia (loss of cuticles with inflammation and infection of nail folds) occurs commonly in association with wet work (Fig. 228).

Management

Management of the underlying eczema, especially around nail folds. Protection from trauma and wet work. Microbiology of nail fold with appropriate treatment of any secondary infection.

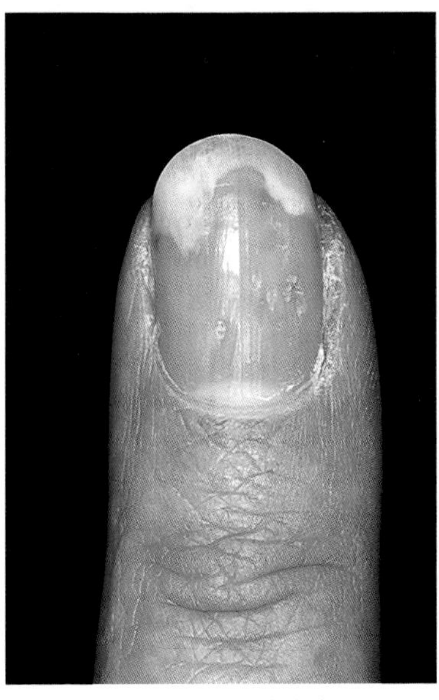

Fig. 225 Pitting and onycholysis (psoriasis).

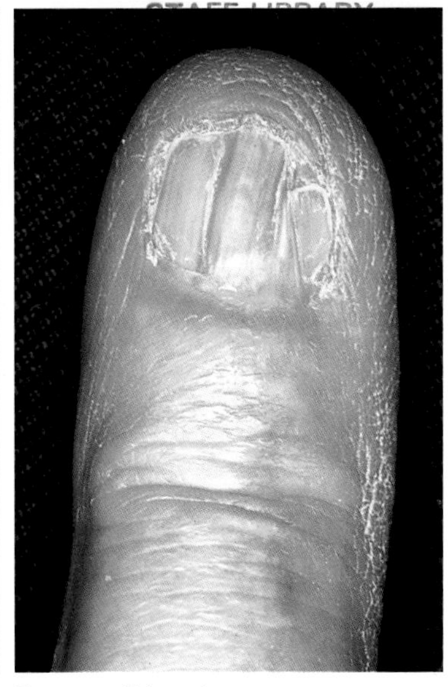

Fig. 226 Lichen planus.

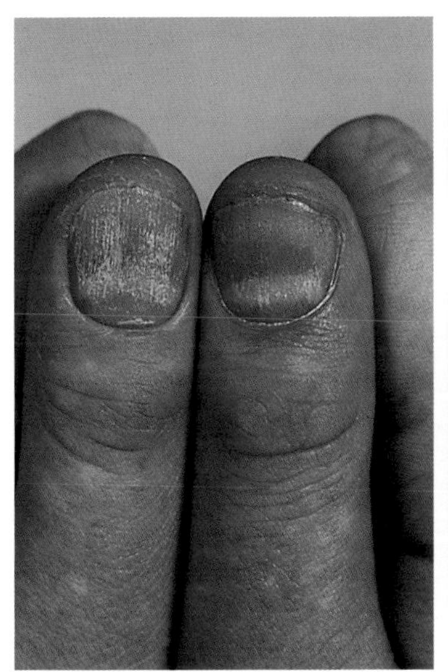

Fig. 227 Fine pitting as seen in alopecia areata and twenty-nail dystrophy.

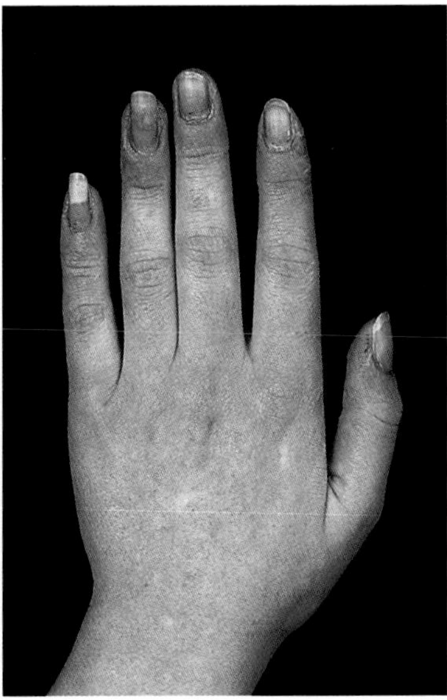

Fig. 228 Chronic paronychia.

40 Hair

Alopecia areata

Aetiology

An organ-specific autoimmune disease.

Clinical features

Characterized by sudden hair loss in discrete, discoid patches (Fig. 229). Spontaneous regrowth often occurs in those with limited disease, although the new hair may initially be white. The condition occasionally progresses to involve the whole scalp (Fig. 230) or body. At the periphery of patches, diagnostic exclamation mark hairs are seen (Fig. 231). There may be associated fine pitting of the nails.

Management

Reassurance and wait for spontaneous regrowth. Topical or intralesional steroids, topical irritants (e.g. dithranol), ultraviolet light/PUVA and contact sensitization may help. Topical 2% minoxidil solution may help those with localized patches.

Scarring alopecia

Aetiology

A result of destruction of hair follicles in, for example, discoid lupus erythematosus, lichen planus, scleroderma, burns, infections and radiodermatitis.

Clinical features

Atrophic scalp with absent hair follicles. Once hair is lost regrowth never occurs.

Management

Treatment of the underlying condition; wig if extensive.

Male pattern baldness (androgenic alopecia)

Aetiology

Genetically determined, androgen-sensitive pattern of hair loss.

Clinical features

Mainly affects men with early bi-temporal recession and loss of hair from vertex (Fig. 232), progressing to more extensive patterns of baldness.

Management

None. Topical 2%–5% minoxidil may reduce the loss or stimulate some hair gain. Finasteride, 1 mg per day. Hair transplant surgery.

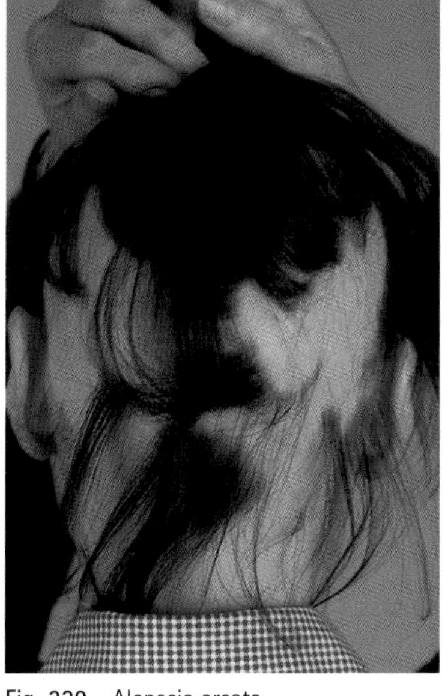

Fig. 229 Alopecia areata.

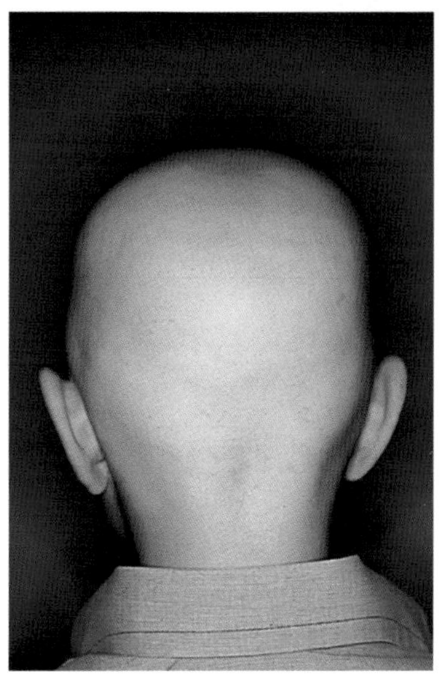

Fig. 230 Alopecia totalis.

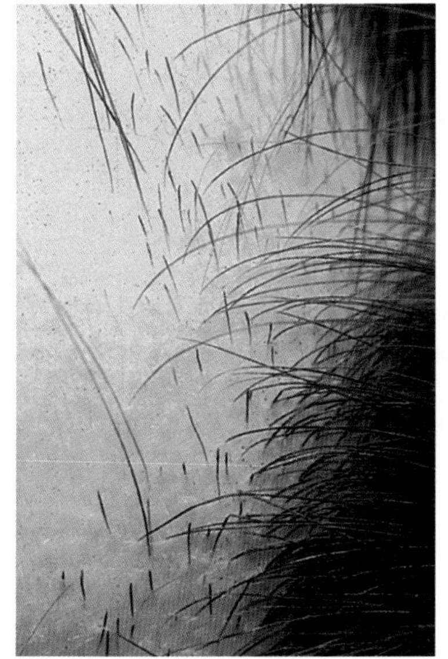

Fig. 231 Exclamation mark hairs in active alopecia areata.

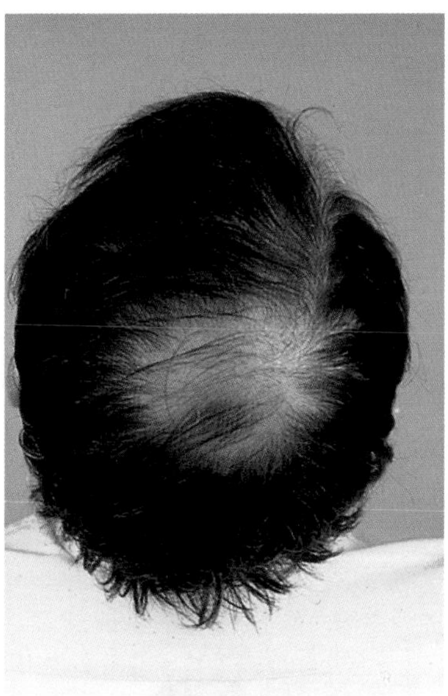

Fig. 232 Bi-temporal recession and early androgenetic hair loss from vertex.

Questions

1. A 12-year-old boy had brown macules on the lips, in the oral cavity and on the extremities, which had been present since infancy.

a. What is the most likely diagnosis?
b. What is the recognized mode of inheritance?
c. What are the possible associated gastrointestinal complications?

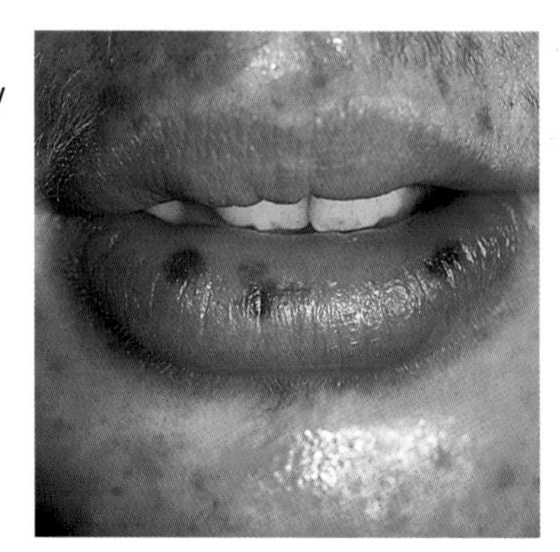

2. Three different patients had the dermatological appearances shown in (a), (b), and (c).

a. What three clinical signs are demonstrated in photographs (a), (b), (c)?
b. What is the unifying diagnosis and mode of inheritance?
c. List other clinical findings that may be observed in this condition.

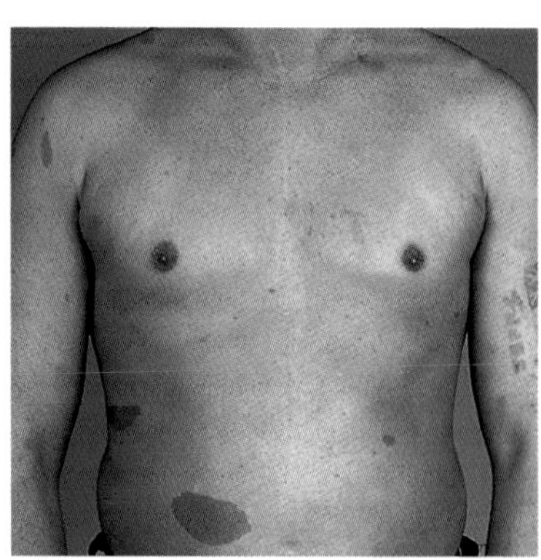

2(a)

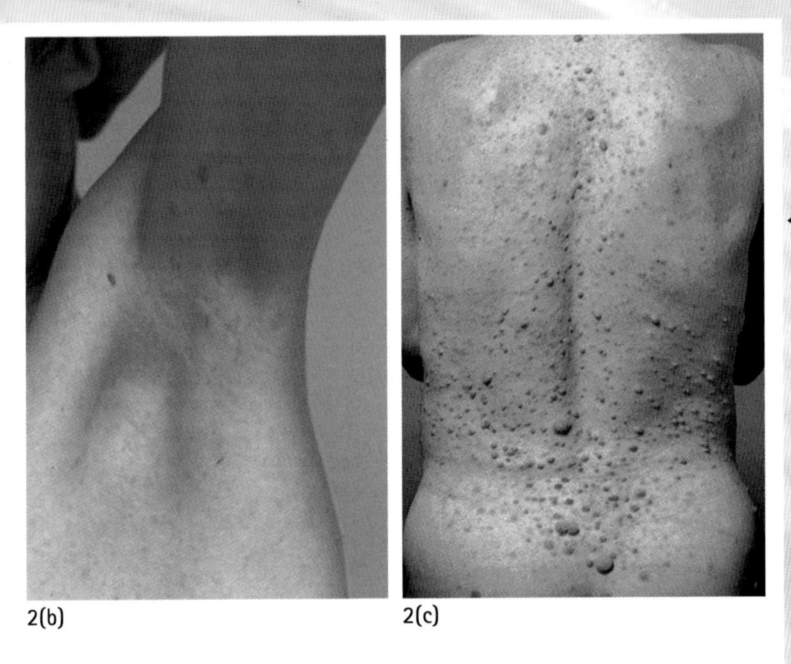

2(b) 2(c)

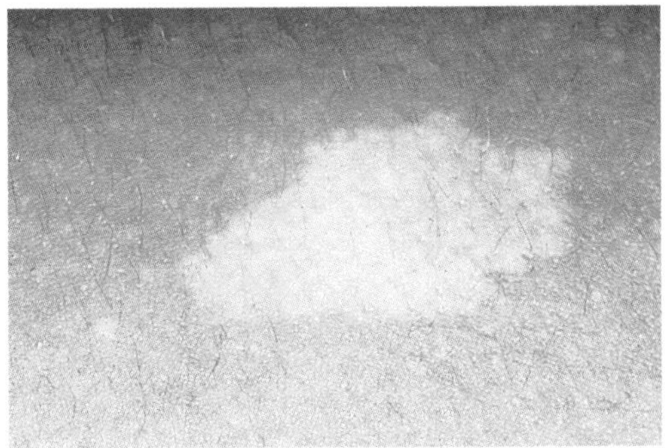

3(a)

3. This 10-year-old girl presented with seizures and developmental delay.

a. What three clinical signs are demonstrated in photographs (a), (b), (c)?
b. What is the unifying diagnosis and mode of inheritance?

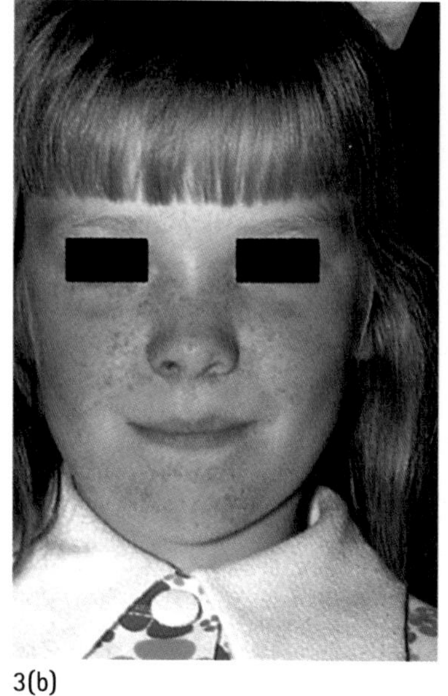

3(b)

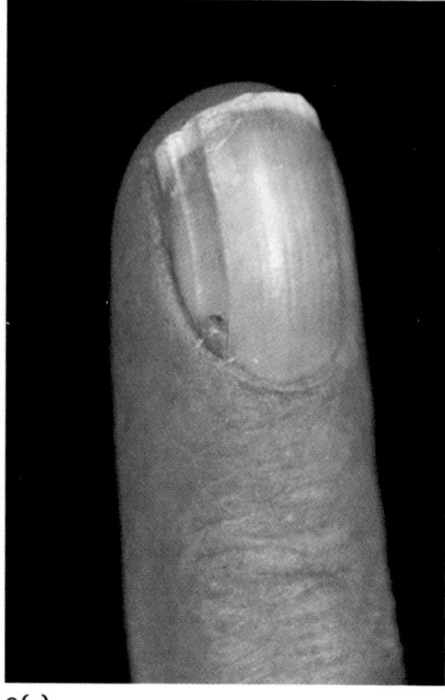

3(c)

4. Three separate patients had the features shown in (a), (b), and (c).

a. What three clinical signs are demonstrated in photographs (a), (b), (c)?
b. What is the unifying diagnosis?
c. List other important clinical complications that may be seen.

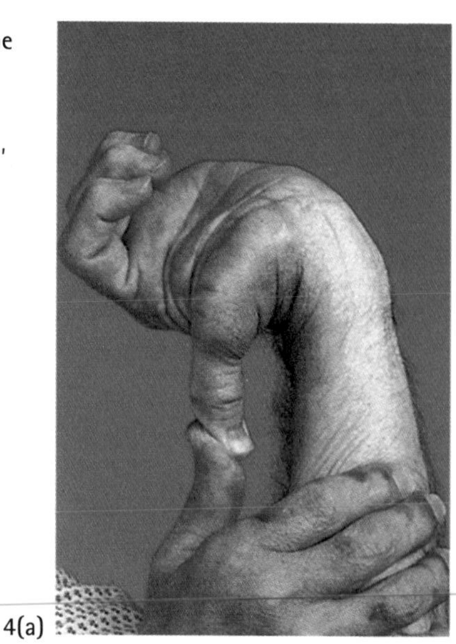

4(a)

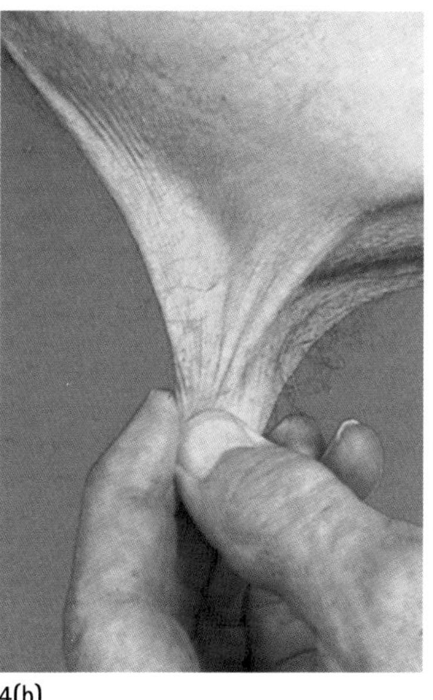

4(b)

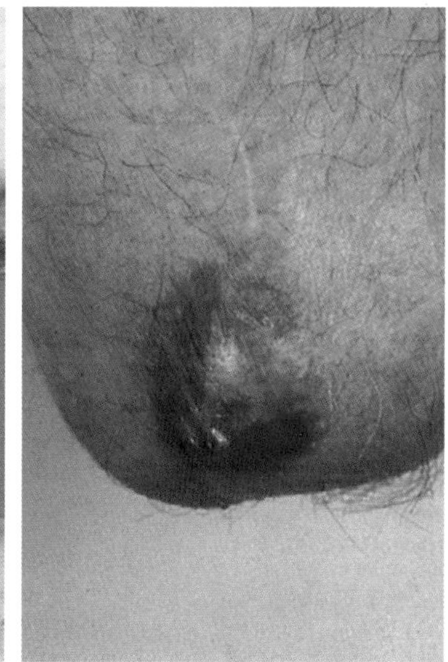

4(c)

5. This asymptomatic 20-year-old patient presented with this appearance on her neck, axillae and antecubital fossae.

a. What clinical sign is demonstrated?
b. What is the diagnosis?
c. What may be seen on fundoscopic examination?
d. What clinical complications may occur, and what might you advise this patient?

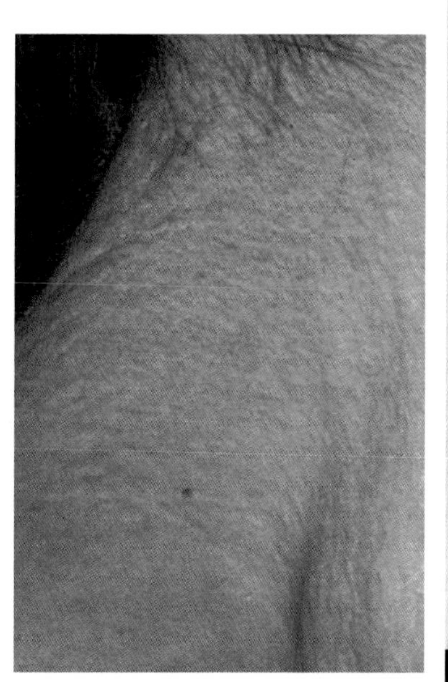

6. This elderly man presented with widespread dry skin.

a. In what group of heterogeneous disorders does the condition belong?
b. List the various possible causes and medical associations.

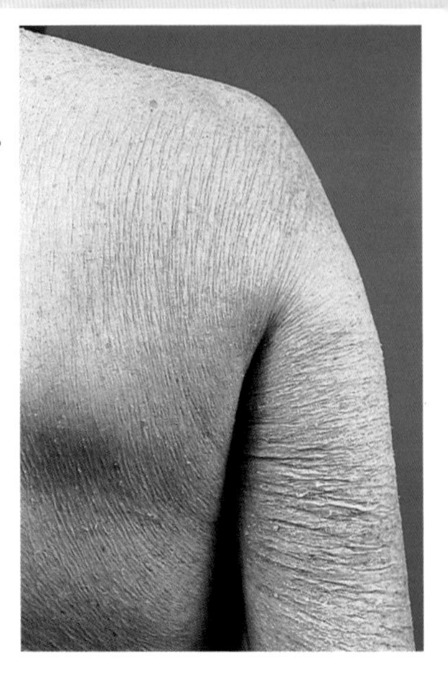

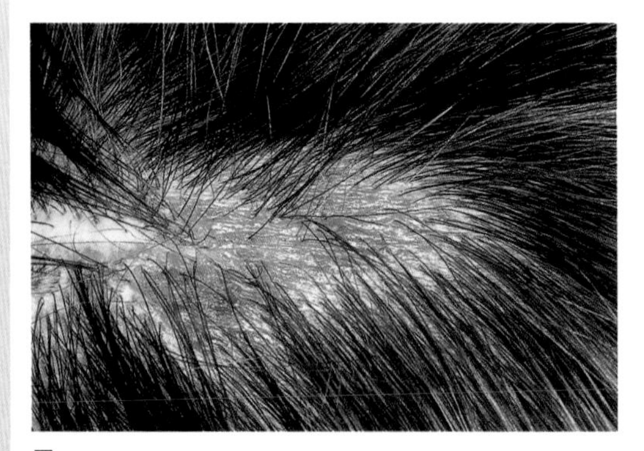

7. This scalp lesion has been present since birth.

a. What is the likely diagnosis?
b. What is the prognosis?
c. What are the management options?

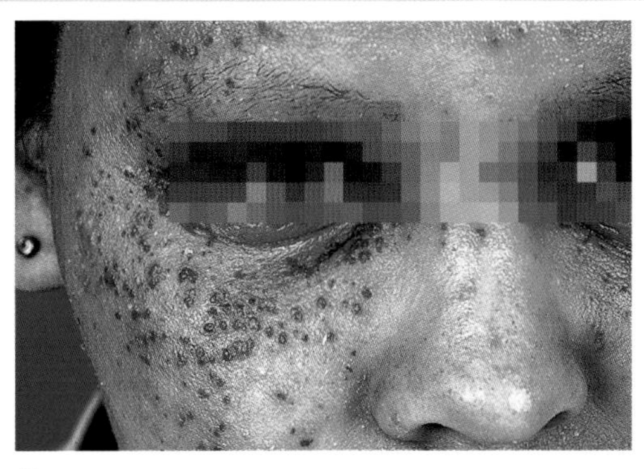

8. This patient with long-standing atopic eczema presented with fever, malaise and a painful rash.

a. What is the diagnosis?
b. What is the classical clinical sign?

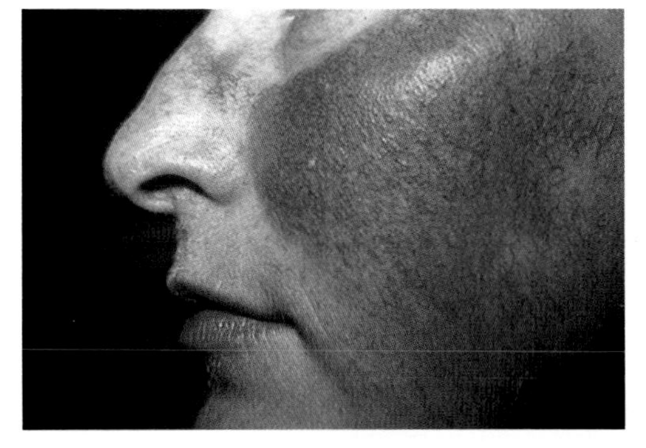

9. This patient has been treated in the past for chronic atopic dermatitis.

a. What are the physical signs demonstrated in these photographs?
b. What is the most likely cause?

10. This patient with flu-like symptoms developed a solitary annular rash after returning from a camping trip in the New Forest.

a. What is the diagnosis?
b. What is the cause?
c. How is the early disease best treated?

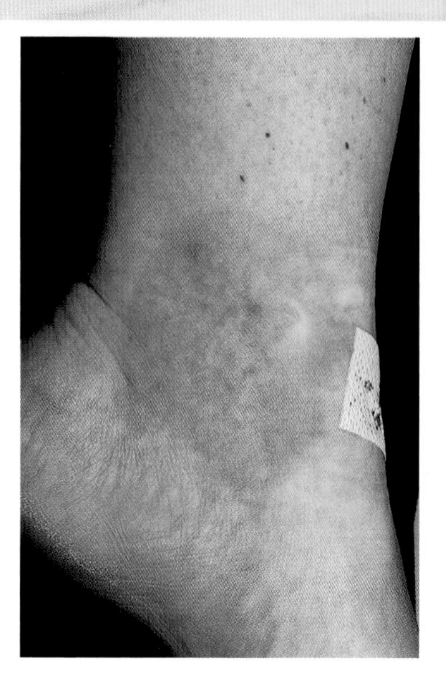

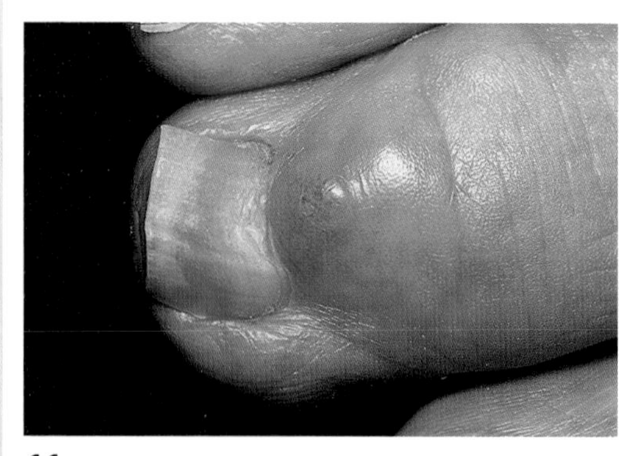

11. This lady presented with an asymptomatic translucent cystic nodule at the nail base.

a. What is the diagnosis?
b. What complications can occur?
c. What treatment may be offered?

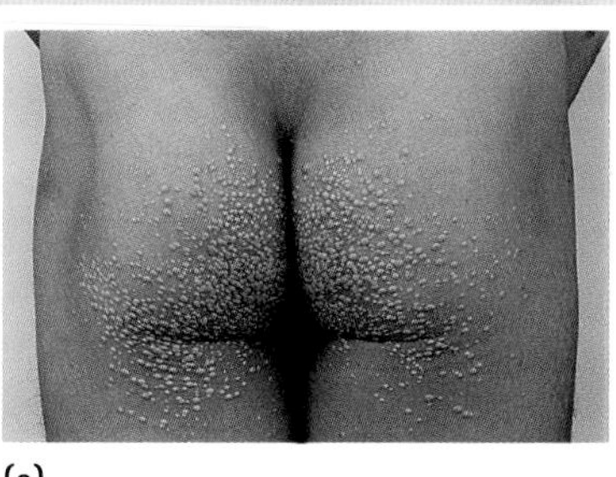

(a)

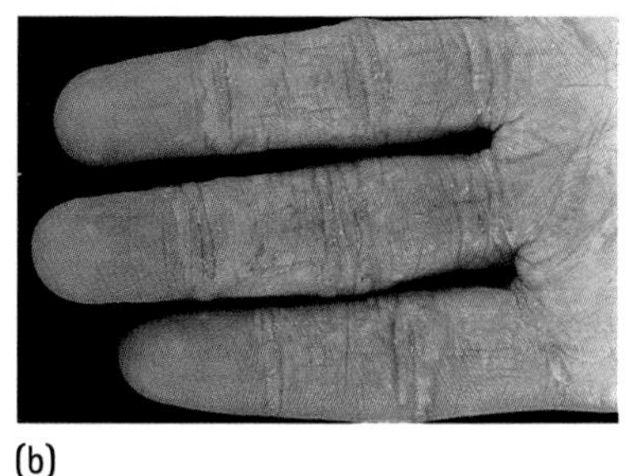

(b)

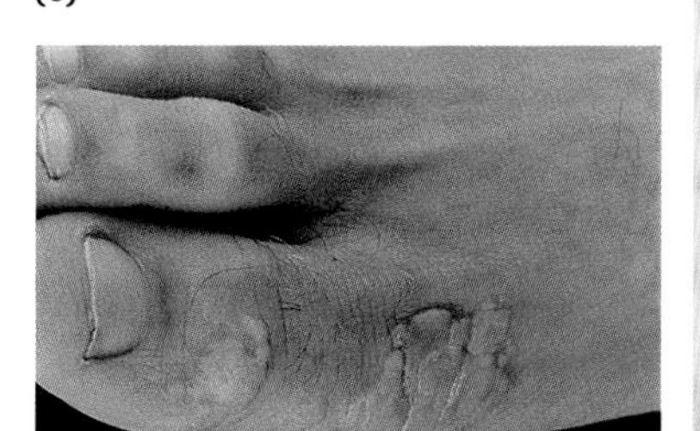

(c)

12. This patient presented with mild jaundice and asymptomatic yellowish papules on the knees, buttocks and palms. More nodular lesions were present on his feet and elbows.

a. What is the likely diagnosis?
b. What biochemical tests would you arrange?
c. What serious acute complication can occur?

13. This patient presented with weight loss and an extensively pigmented rash in the axillae and groin flexures, which had developed over the past few months.

a. What is the most likely diagnosis?
b. What is the likely cause?

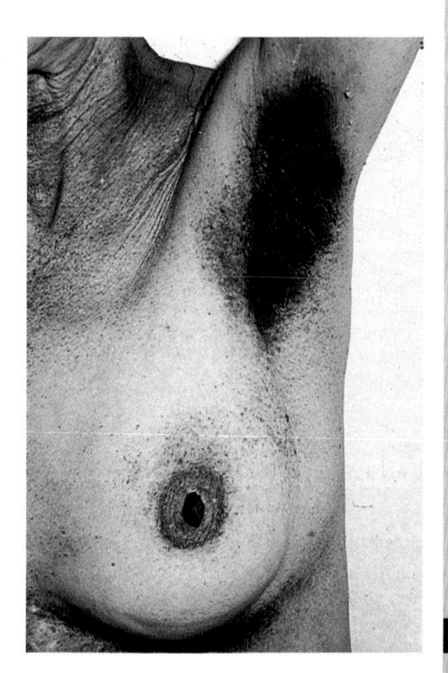

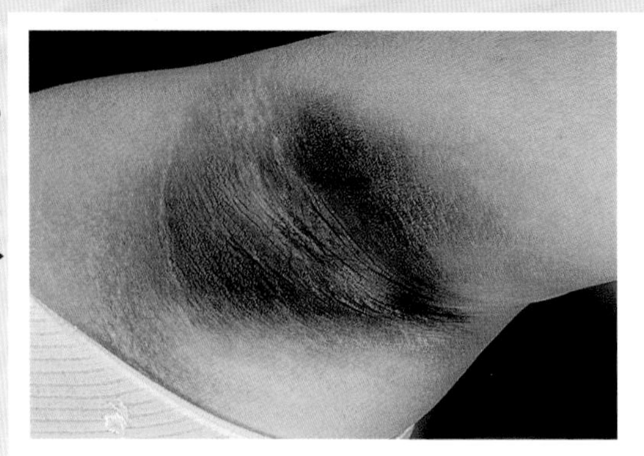

14. This 13-year-old obese girl presented with this asymptomatic appearance around her axillae and neck.

a. What is the likely diagnosis?
b. What conditions may be associated with it?

15. This patient, who had recently been treated for internal malignancy, presented with recurrent inflammation over some of his forearm veins.

a. What is the diagnosis?
b. What other skin signs have been reported as reliable signs of internal malignancy?

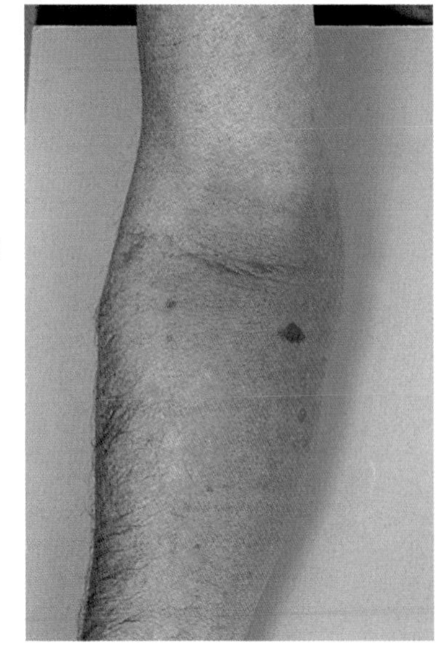

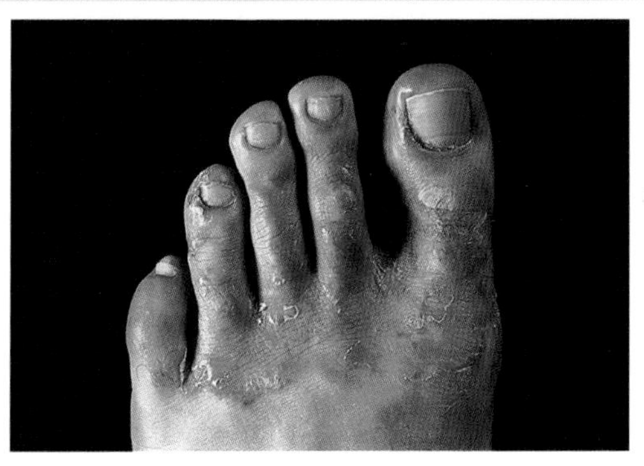

16. This patient had been applying a topical corticosteroid to his foot for presumed eczema, and the rash got worse after initial improvement.

a. What are the physical signs, and what investigation should be performed?
b. What is the diagnosis?
c. What is the treatment?

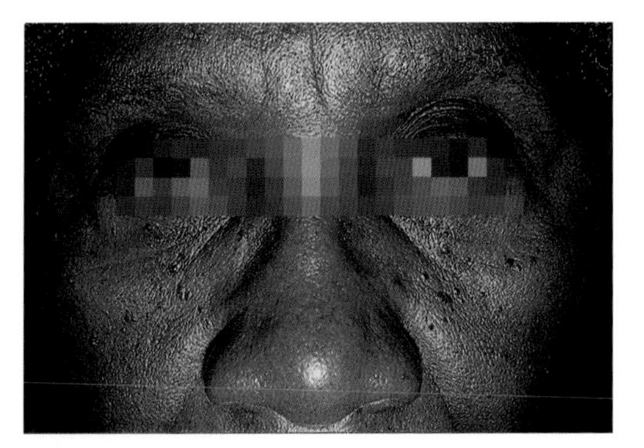

17. This female patient was concerned about the cosmetic appearance of these long-standing hyperpigmented papules.

a. What is the diagnosis?
b. How should they be treated?

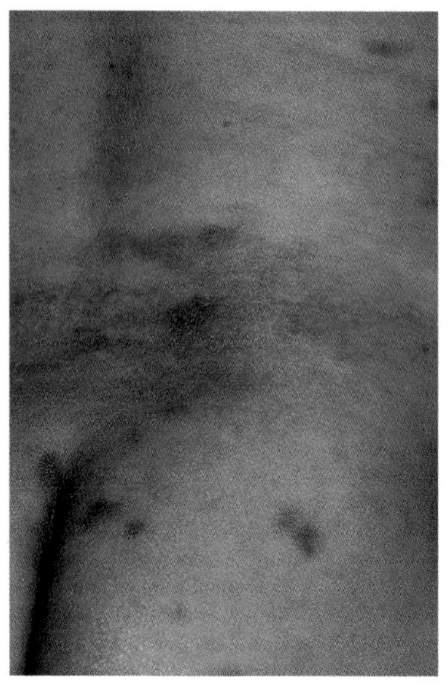

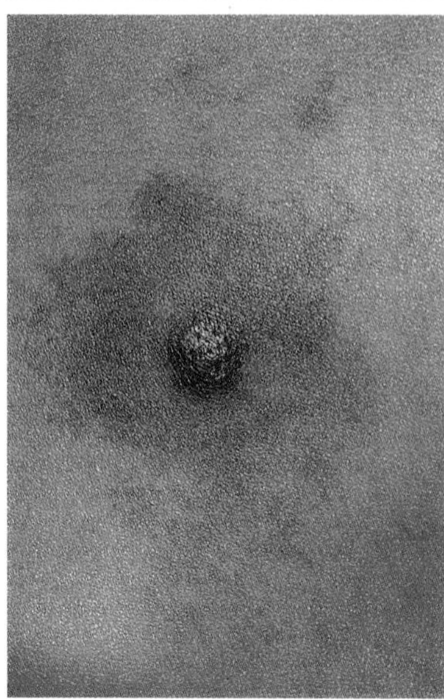

18. This child presented with pruritic brown macular patches over the trunk, which become red and swollen after rubbing.

a. What is the diagnosis?
b. What is the name of the sign that indicates urtication or blistering if the lesions are rubbed?
c. What is the treatment?

19. This patient presented with a large number of irregular moles. There is a family history of melanoma.

a. What is the most likely diagnosis?
b. What is its clinical importance?
c. What advice would you give the patient?

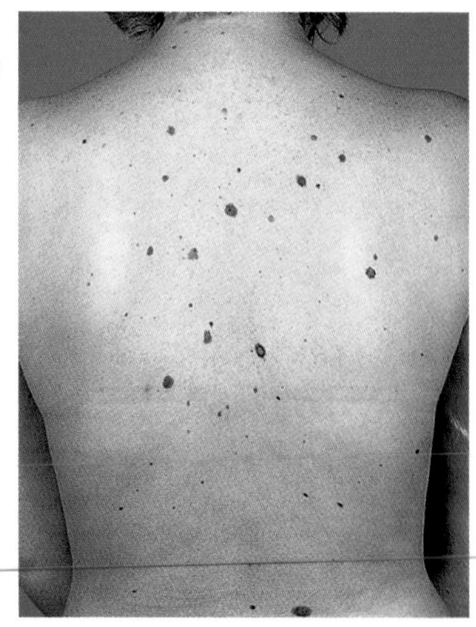

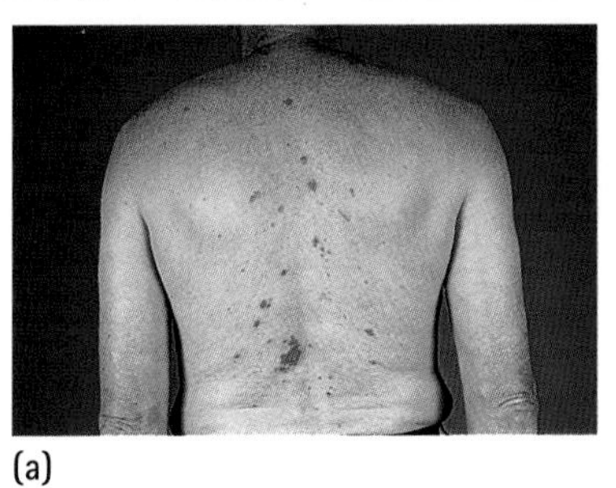
(a)

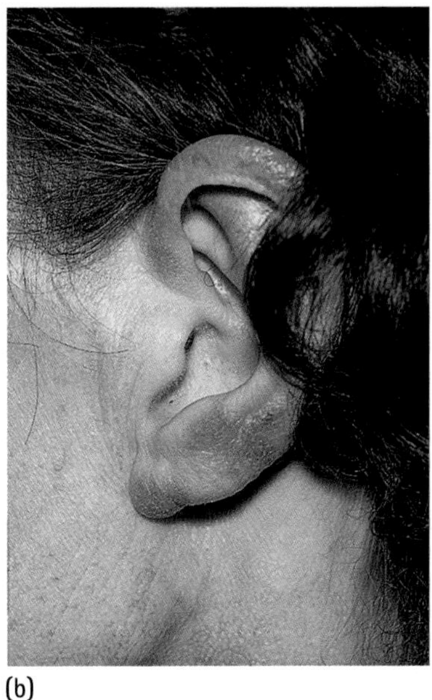
(b)

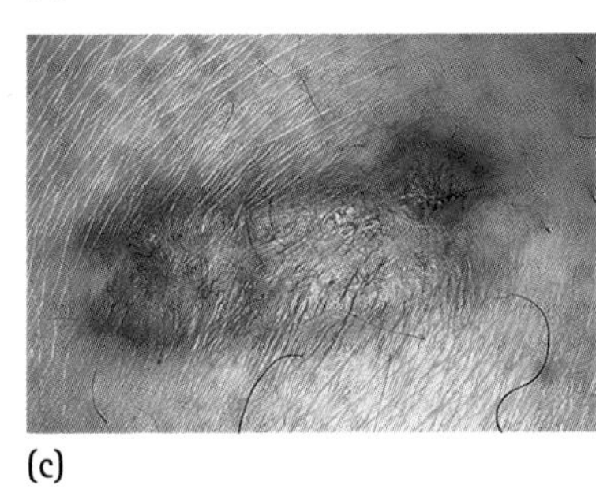
(c)

20. This woman with arthralgia presented with asymptomatic erythematous papules and plaques on skin, dusky erythema of nose and ears and a reaction in an old scar.

a. What are the specific diagnoses that are demonstrated in the three illustrations (a), (b), (c)?

b. What further diagnostic investigations would you consider and why?

c. When would systemic treatment be indicated?

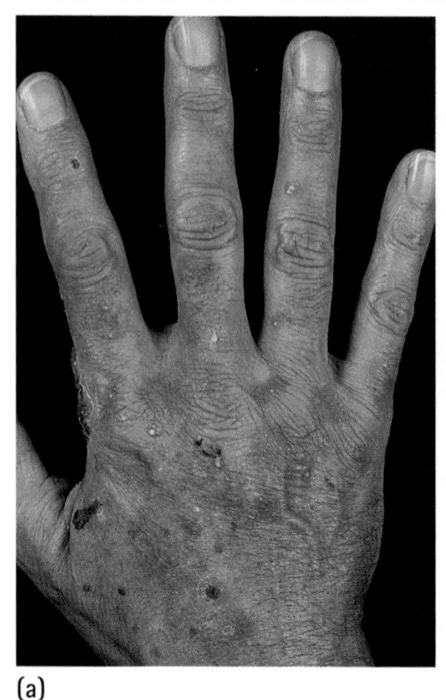

(a)

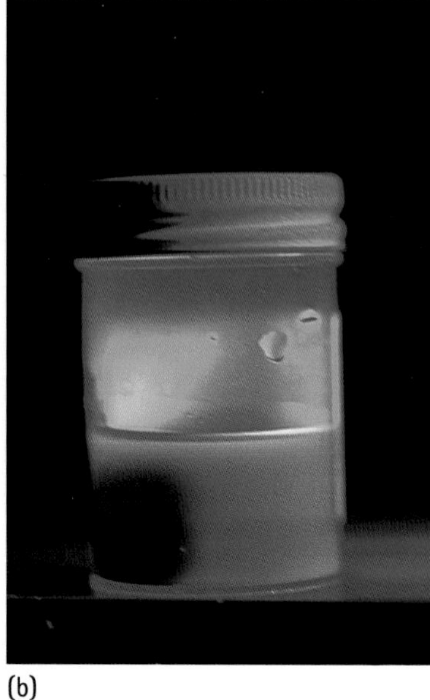

(b)

21. A man presents with fragility and blistering of the skin of his hands and with diffuse hyperpigmentation, especially of exposed sites. Wood's light examination of his urine is shown in photograph (b).

a What three clinical signs are shown?
b. What are the two clinical diagnoses?
c. How can the pigmentation be related to his other skin changes?
d. How would you treat this man?

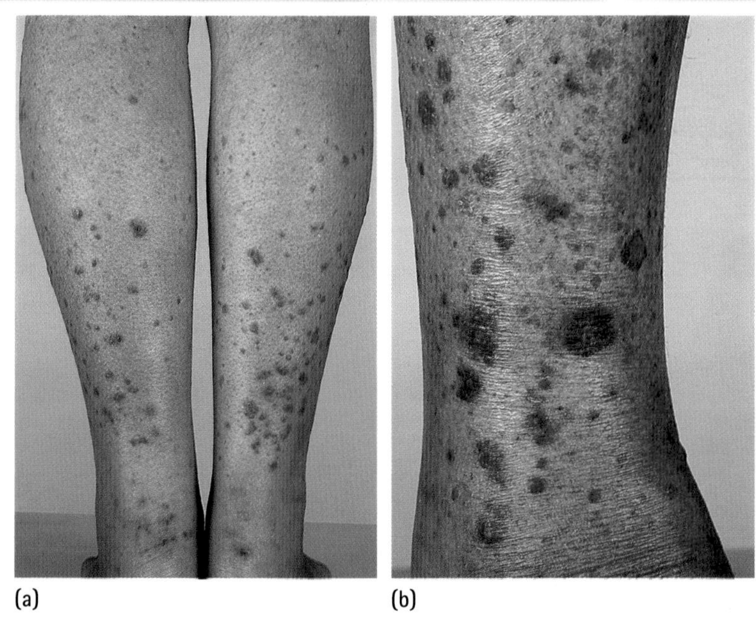

(a) (b)

22. This lady presented with a 2-week history of this rash on her legs and arthralgia.

a. What clinical features and diagnosis are shown in photographs (a) and (b)?
b. What investigation is mandatory?
c. What other investigations would you consider?
d. What are the treatment options?

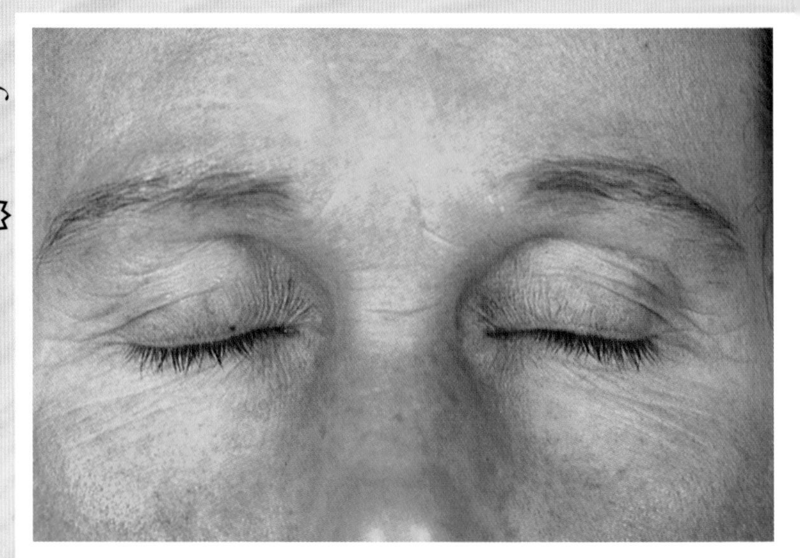

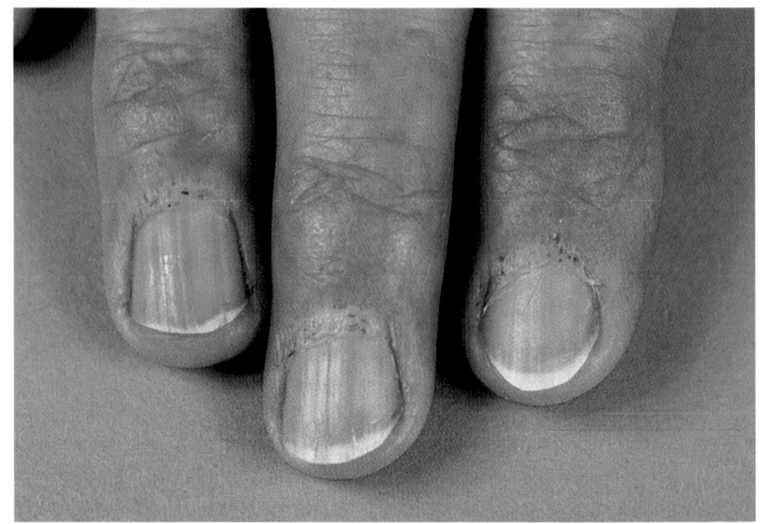

23. This patient presented with erythema of her face, upper chest and dorsa of hands.

a. What clinical findings are shown in the figures?
b. What is the likely diagnosis, and what other abnormal physical findings would you expect to find?
c. What investigations would you undertake, and why?

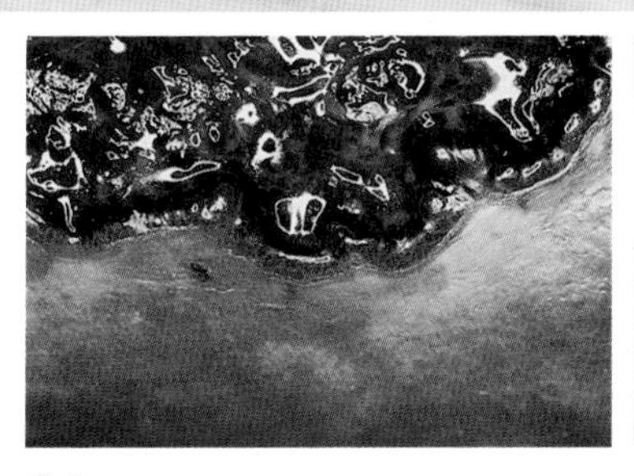

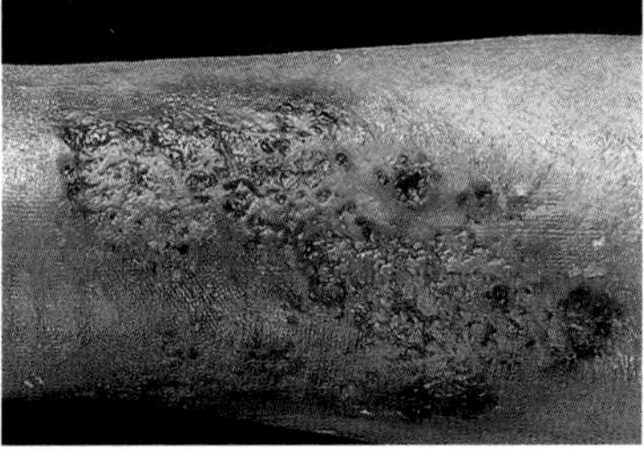

24. This patient developed recurrent ulcers on various parts of the body, showing healing with cribriform scarring.

a. What is the diagnosis?
b. List possible causes.

25. This girl suffers from recurrent painful, dusky erythematous areas on the backs of her heels, feet, and hands, particularly during the winter months.

a. What is the diagnosis?
b. What investigations are required?
c. What is the correct management?

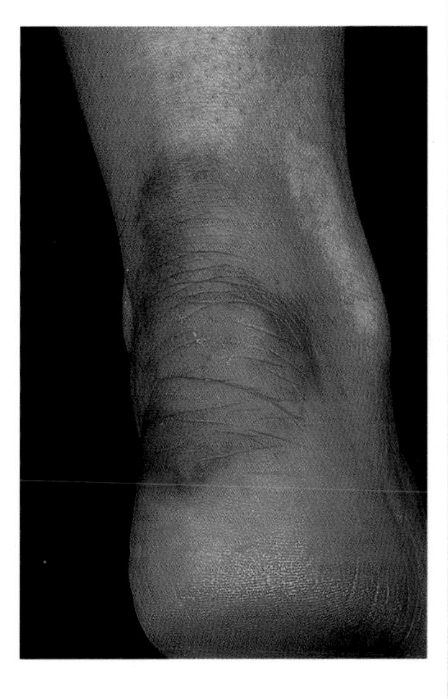

(a) (b)

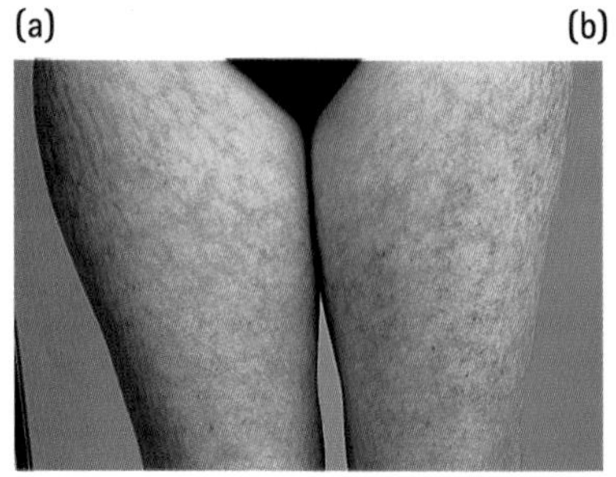

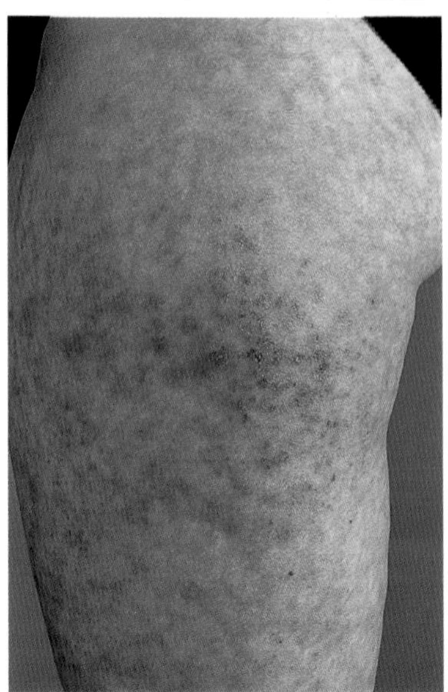

26. This young woman complained of a rash on her thighs, more noticeable during the winter months (a) and associated with tender indurated erythema (b). She is a keen horse rider and reported that her fingers and feet change colour after exposure to the cold and that she sometimes develops ulcers on the fingertips and toes.

a. What skin changes are shown in each of the photographs (a) and (b)?
b. List the possible medical associations of the condition in (a).

(a) (b)

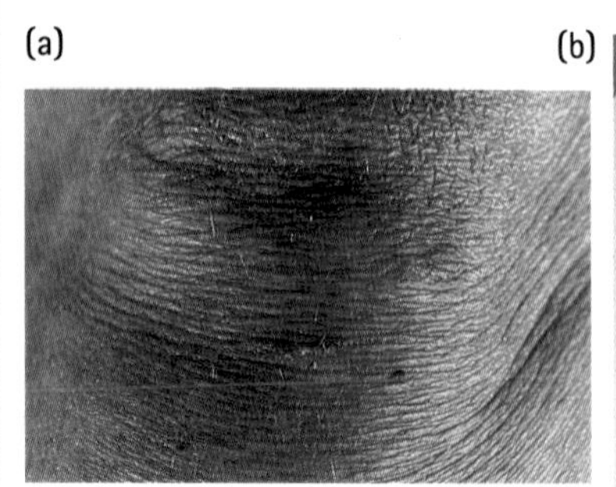

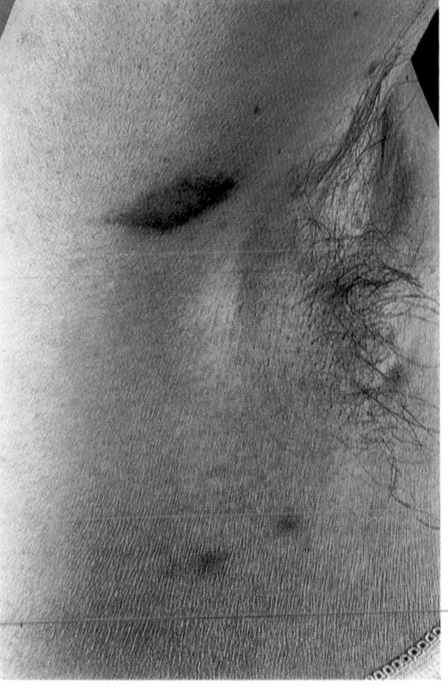

27. This young woman has a very pruritic rash which is worse at night.

a. What clinical signs are shown in photographs (a) and (b)?
b. What additional history should you try to elicit?
c. Name four other generalized itchy rashes.

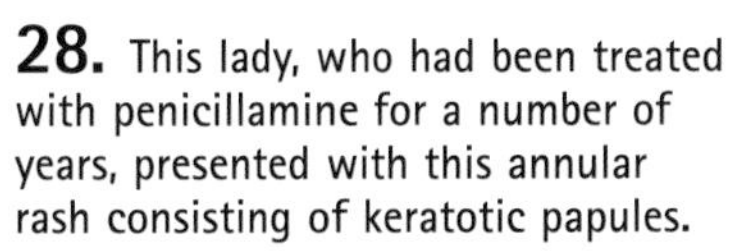

28. This lady, who had been treated with penicillamine for a number of years, presented with this annular rash consisting of keratotic papules.

a. What is the diagnosis?
b. What is the pathogenesis?
c. With what other conditions is this phenomenon associated?
d. What other cutaneous problems have been described with penicillamine.

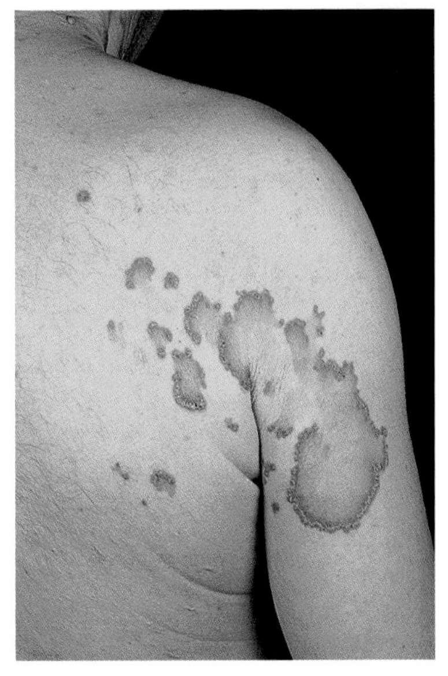

29. This man suffers from dandruff and recurrent crusting and weeping of the skin in and around his ears. He has received repeated applications of topical antibiotics.

a. What is the diagnosis?
b. What investigations may be relevant?
c. What would be appropriate initial treatment?

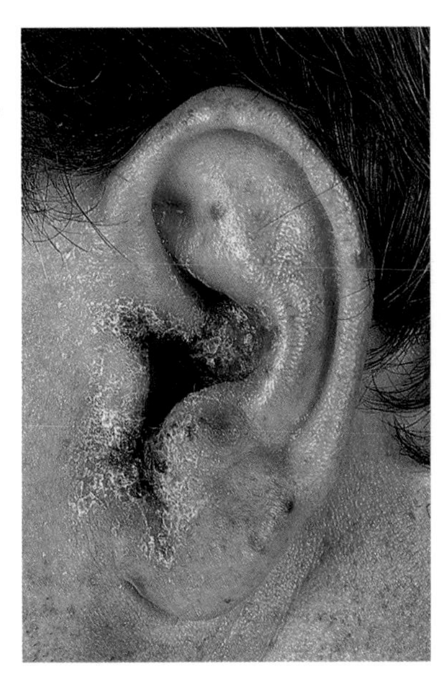

30. An elderly lady, who has previously suffered with leg ulcers and had multiple hip surgery procedures in the past, presents with the leg shown here.

a What clinical findings, excluding the surgical scar, are shown?
b. What is the underlying cause of these changes?

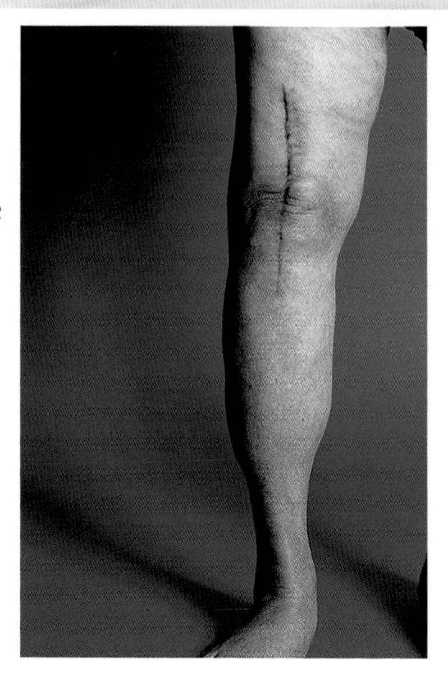

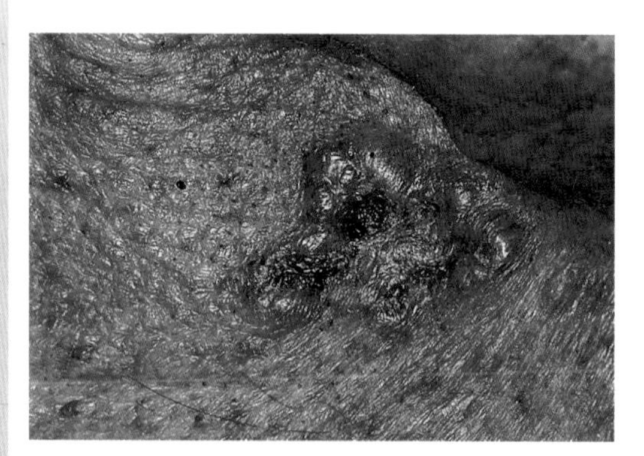

31. An elderly man has this lesion on his face, present for 18 months.

a. What is the diagnosis?
b. What other skin changes can be seen?
c. What is the correct management?

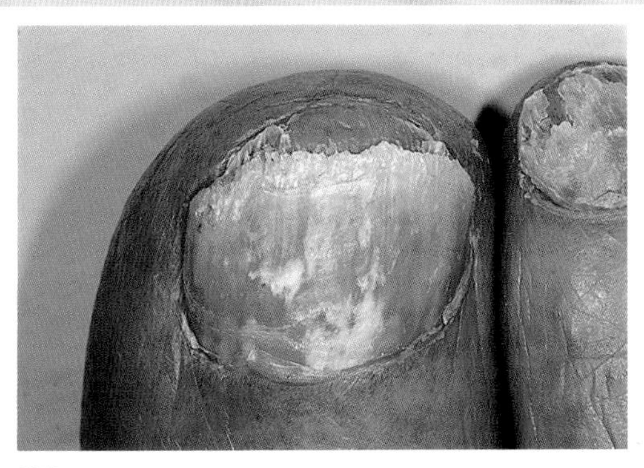

32. This woman has chronic dystrophy of her toenails.

a. What is the most likely diagnosis?
b. What investigations are appropriate?
c. What treatment would you recommend?

33. This man has firm, raised, slightly hyperpigmented nodules and plaques over his shoulders, chest and upper back, present for 2 years.

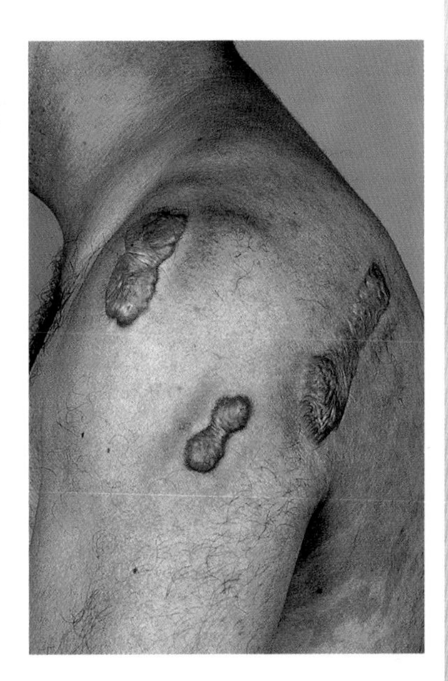

a. What is the diagnosis?
b. What may have caused these lesions?
c. What differentiates these lesions from ordinary scars?
d. What treatment is possible?

34. This elderly man presented with a painful and tender nodule on the rim of his ear, which prevents him from resting his head on his pillow.

a. What is the diagnosis?
b. What is the presumed patho-aetiology?
c. What treatment is possible?

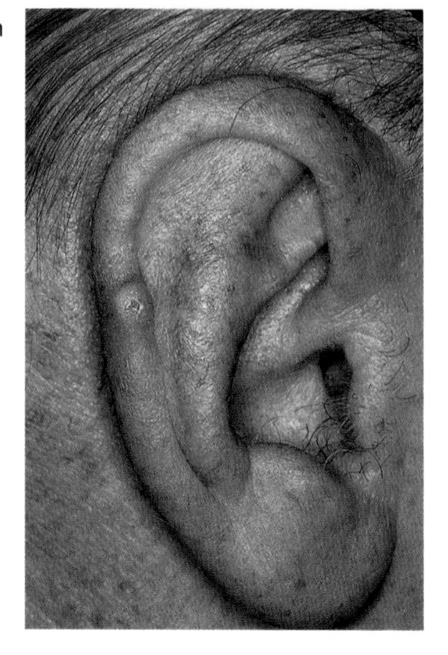

35. This lady was admitted to Accident and Emergency with rigors, high temperature and nausea/ vomiting of sudden onset. Her left lower leg was hot and red. She gives a history of penicillin allergy.

a. What is the diagnosis?
b. What would be an appropriate treatment regimen?
c. What conditions might predispose to it?
d. What complications might occur?

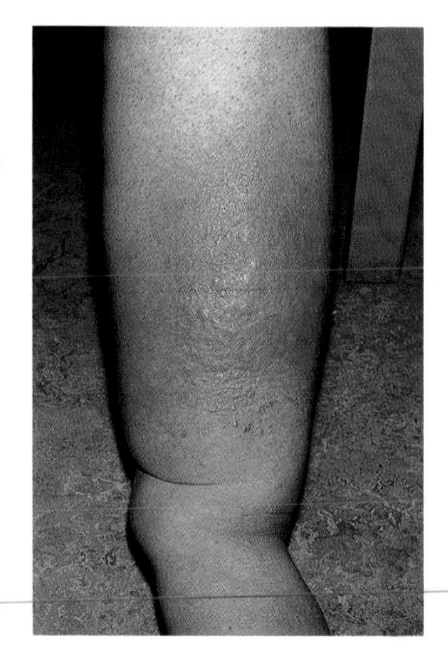

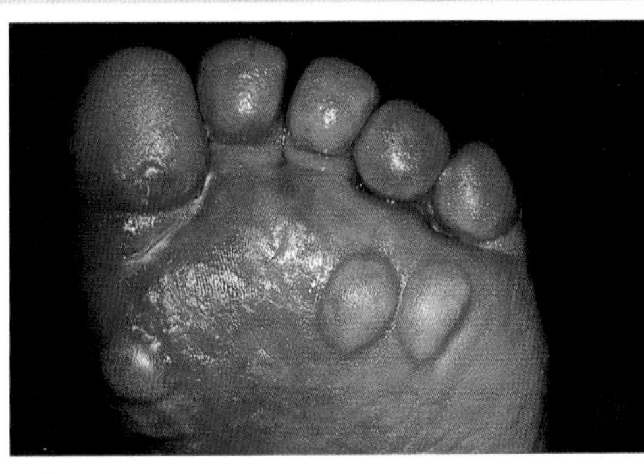

36. A young person has acute blistering of the soles of the feet.

a. What is the diagnosis?
b. What are the possible causes?

37. This man presented with a mostly asymptomatic dry, scaly, well-delineated hyperpigmented rash affecting axillae and groins. The rash fluoresced pink under Wood's light.

a. What is the diagnosis?
b. What is the patho-aetiology?
c. How can the condition be treated?

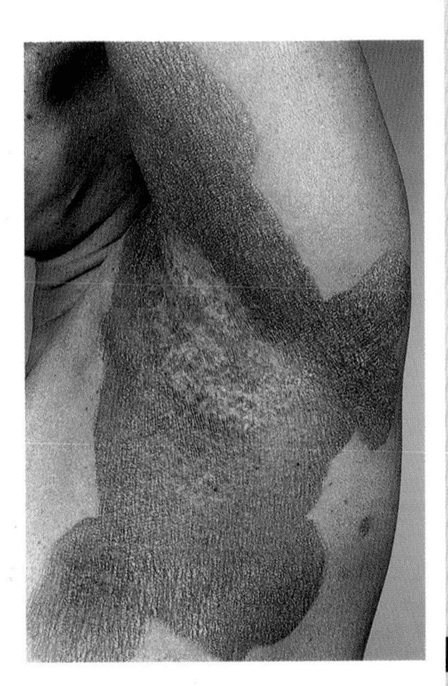

38. This adolescent presented with a widespread rash following penicillin for a chronic sore throat and malaise.

a. What is the probable diagnosis?
b. What further examination or investigations are required?
c. Will it be safe to give penicillin again in later life?

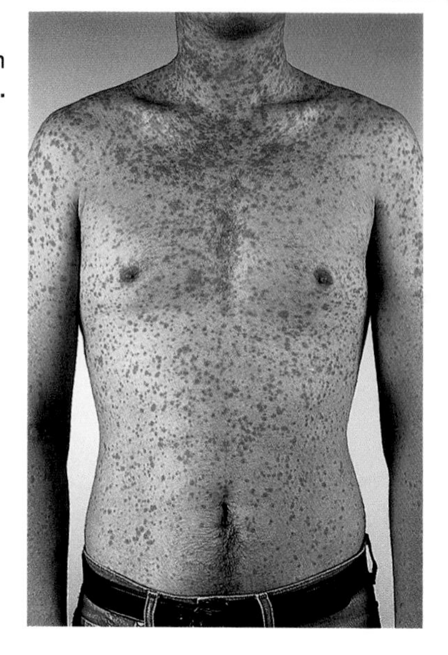

39. This man has had a persistent discharging nodule on the right jaw for several years.

a. What is the diagnosis?
b. What investigation is needed?
c. What is the treatment?

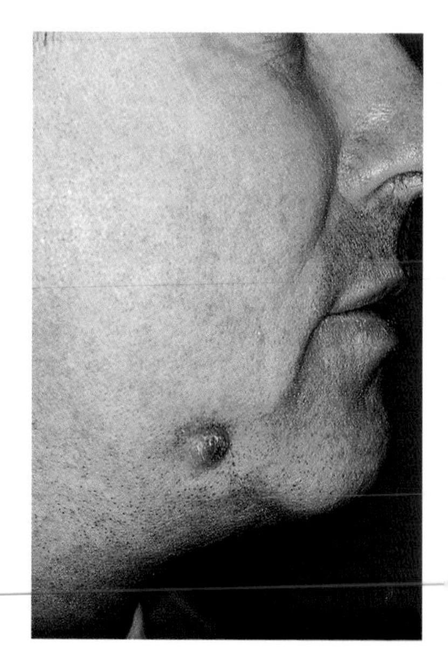

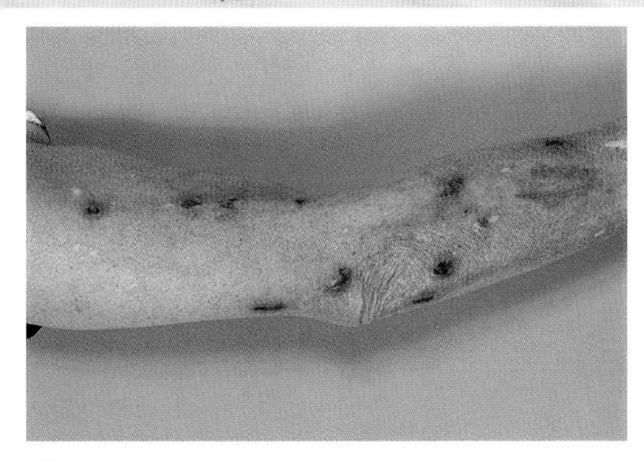

40. This elderly lady has had chronic relapsing itchy nodules on her limbs for several years.

a. What is the most likely diagnosis?
b. What investigations might be appropriate?
c. What possible treatments might be effective?

41. A woman presented with a slowly progressive, velvety, erythematous and slightly pigmented perianal plaque. There was no evidence of any skin disease elsewhere.

a. What is the differential diagnosis?
b. What investigations are necessary?

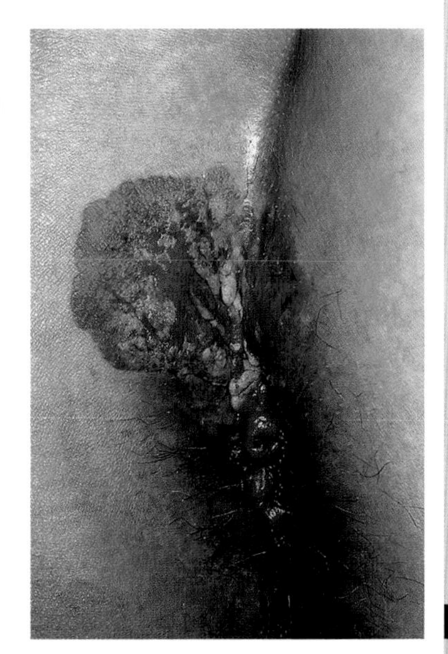

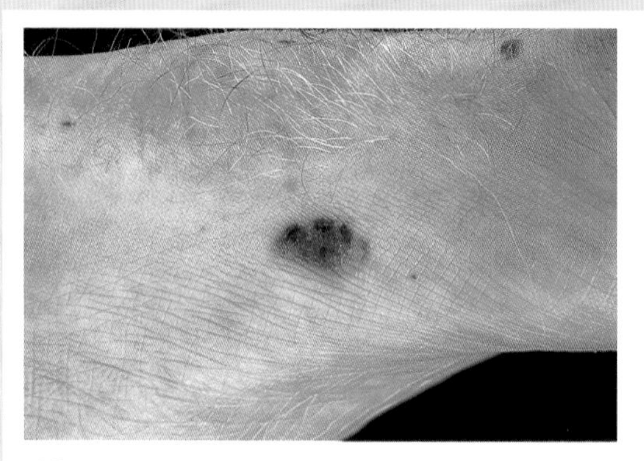

42. This 46-year-old man noticed a changing mole.

a. What clinical features are shown?
b. What is the diagnosis?
c. What is the appropriate management?

43. This young woman has been getting tender red lumps on her legs (and occasionally arms) for the last 6 weeks.

a. What is the diagnosis?
b. What are the possible causes?
c. Name three other types of infection that may cause this reaction.
d. Name some drugs that may be responsible.

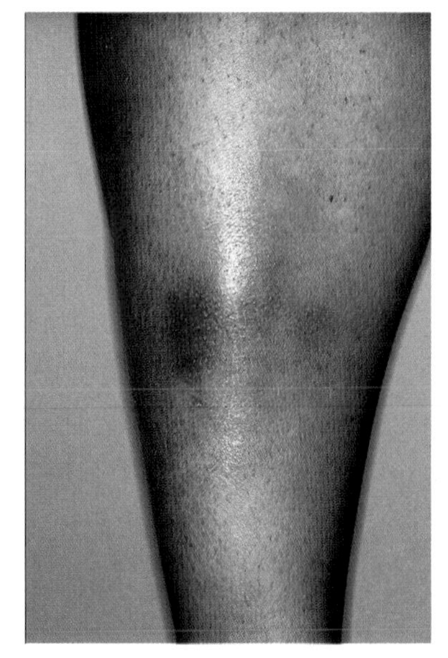

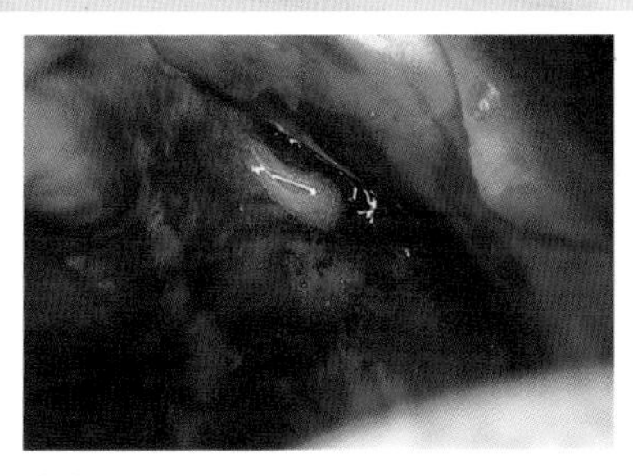
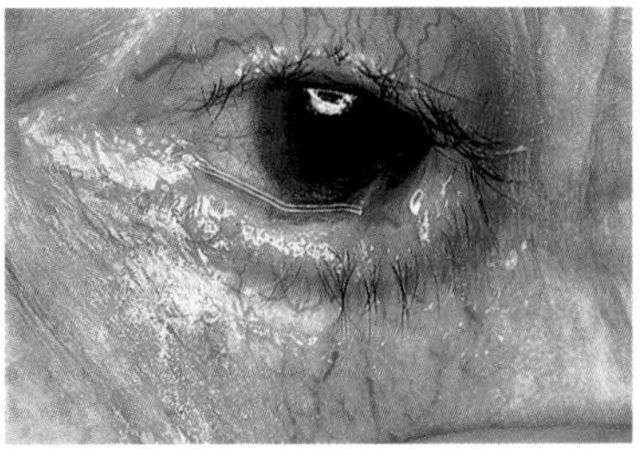

44. This elderly lady presented with sore erosions in the mouth, with this appearance of the eyes and occasional blisters on her head.

a. What is the unifying diagnosis?
b. What other complications may occur?

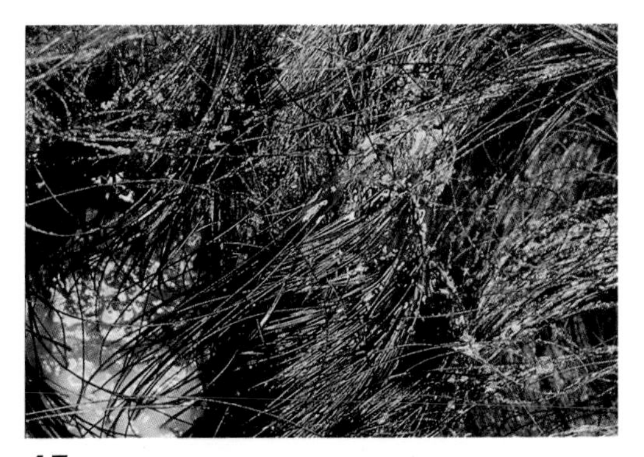

45. This child has an itchy scalp.

a. What is the diagnosis?
b. How would you manage the case?

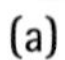

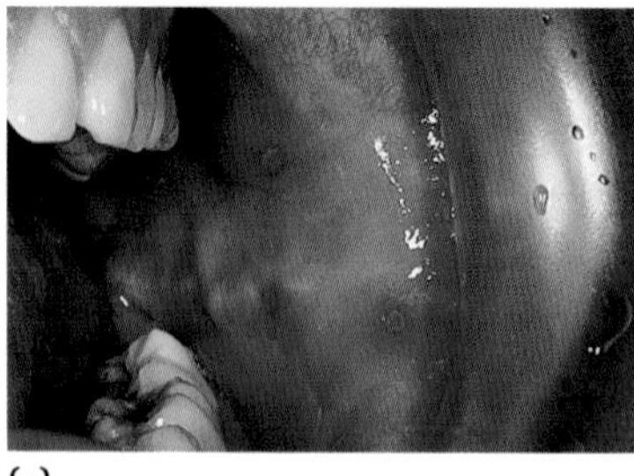

(a)

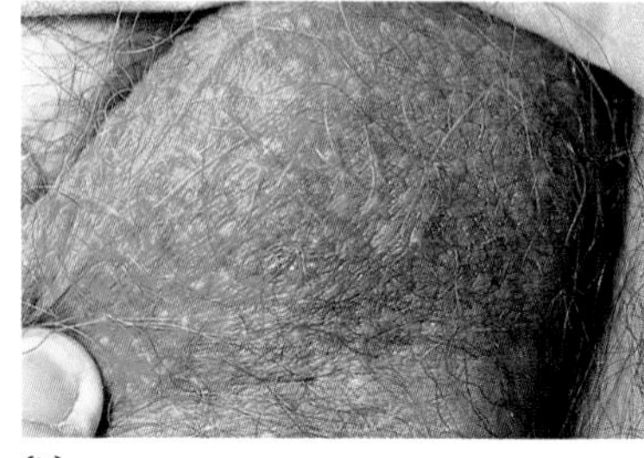

(b)

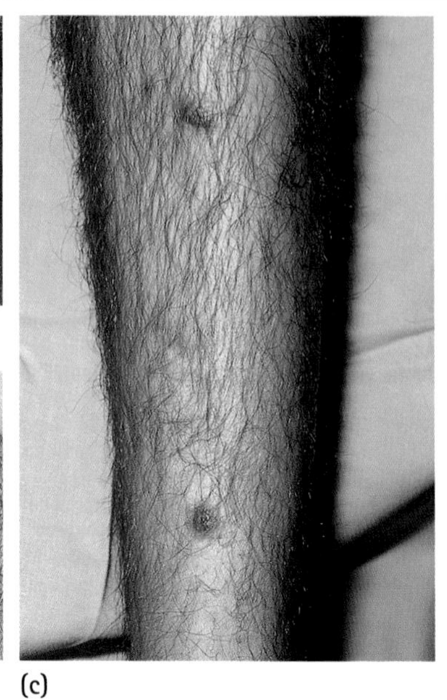

(c)

46. This young man suffers from recurrent painful oro-genital ulceration.

a. What mucocutaneous findings are shown?
b. What other symptoms might you enquire about and why?

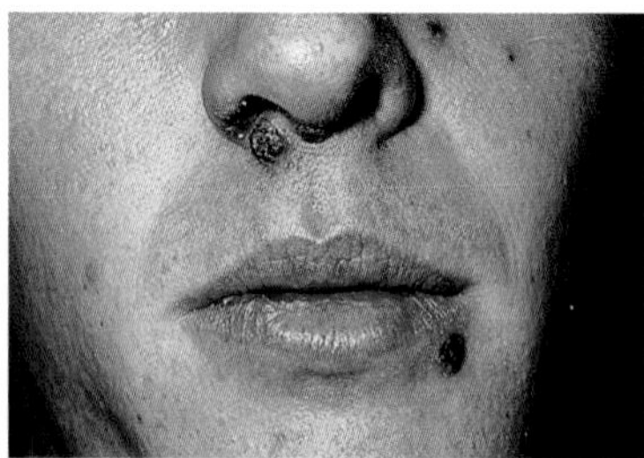

(d)

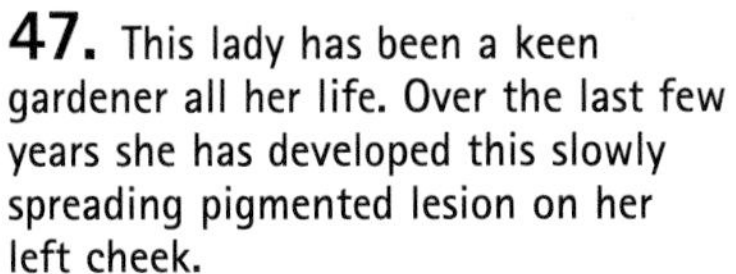

47. This lady has been a keen gardener all her life. Over the last few years she has developed this slowly spreading pigmented lesion on her left cheek.

a. What is the diagnosis?
b. What are the treatment options?

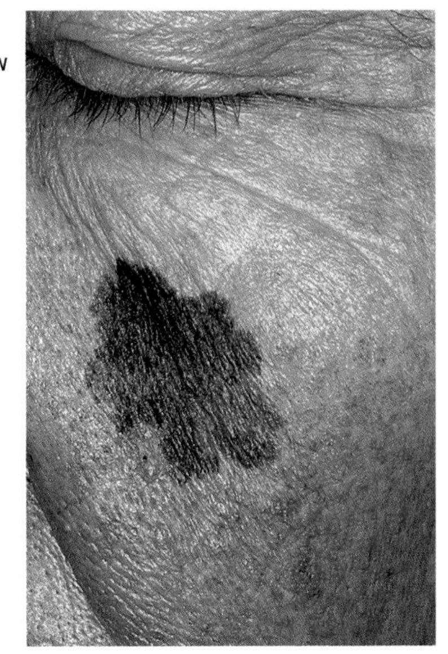

48. This woman developed asymptomatic pigmentation on her forehead, on her cheeks and around her mouth.

a. What is the diagnosis?
b. What are the main patho-aetiological factors?
c. What treatment is possible?

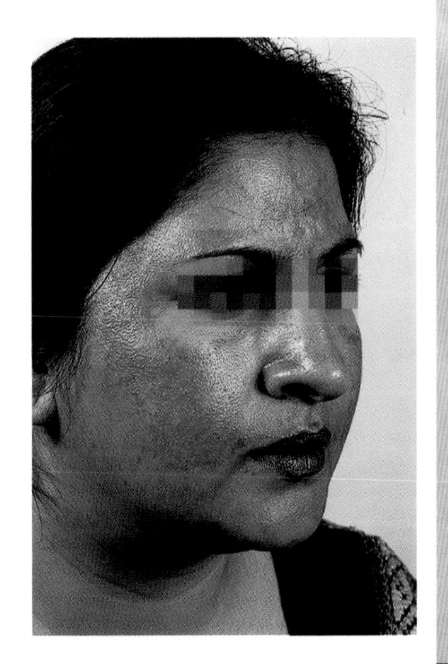

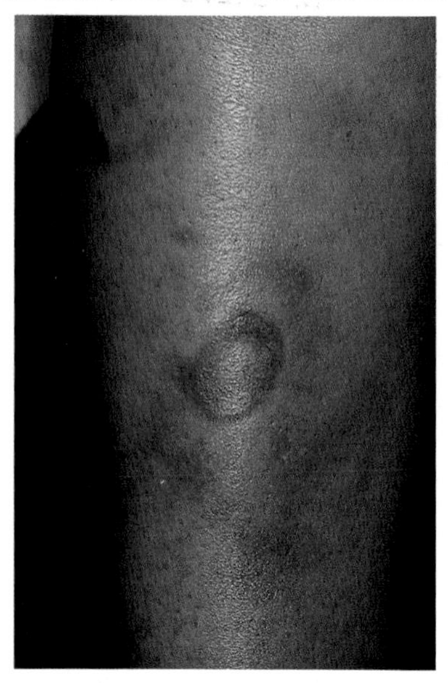

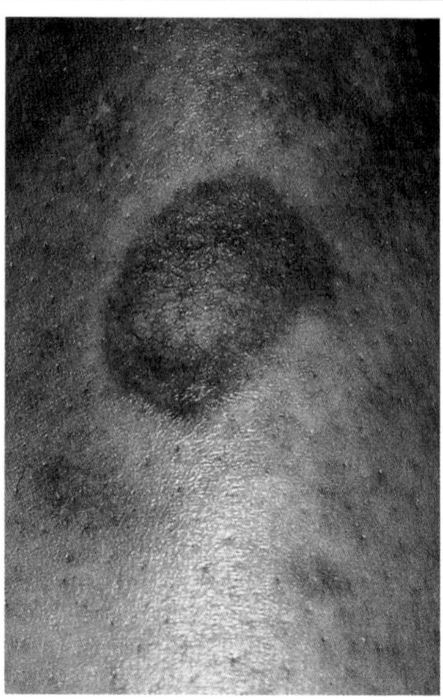

49. This young woman presented with shiny, 'waxy', slightly atrophic reddish-brown plaques on her lower legs for about 2 years.

a. What is the diagnosis?
b. Are there any medical associations?
c. What is the major complication?

50. This young man has noticed these smooth red patches on his tongue. There are no associated symptoms, except when he eats salty, citrus or spicy food.

a. What is the diagnosis?
b. What is the treatment?

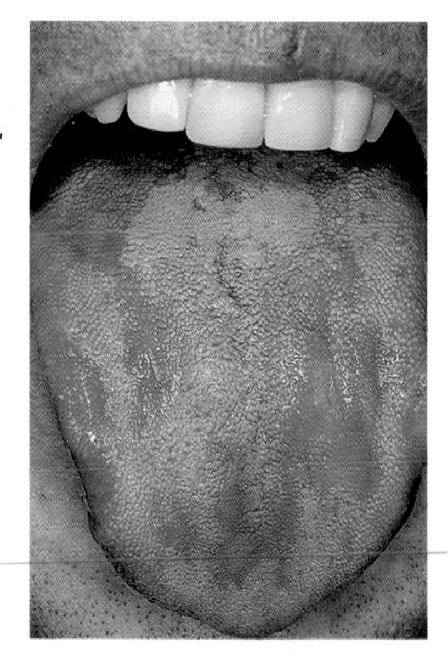

51. This woman had a persistent painless ulcer on the sole of her right foot. She is diabetic with abnormal liver function tests.

a. What is the likely underlying process for the cause of this ulcer?
b. What may be the underlying diseases?

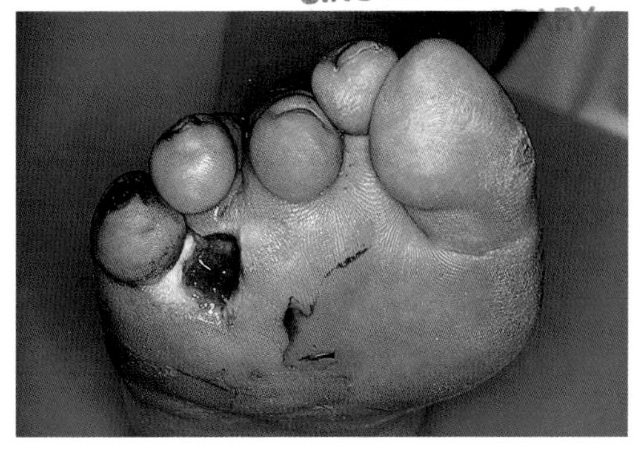

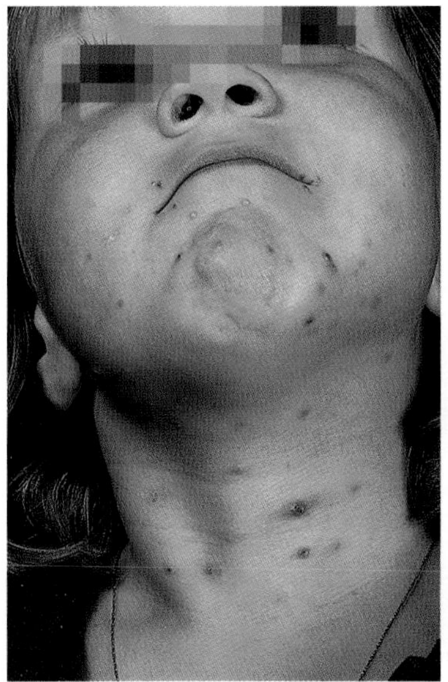

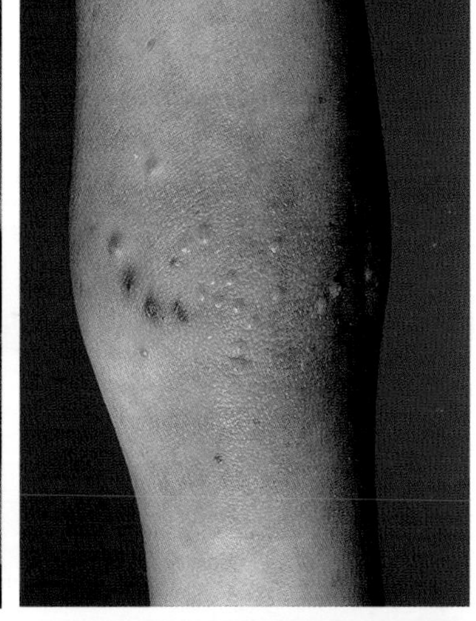

52. An atopic child presented with a spotty rash on her trunk, one of her limbs and her face. The lesions have not persisted, but some new lesions continue to develop and some older lesions healed to leave chickenpox-like scars.

a. What is the diagnosis?
b. How can it be treated?

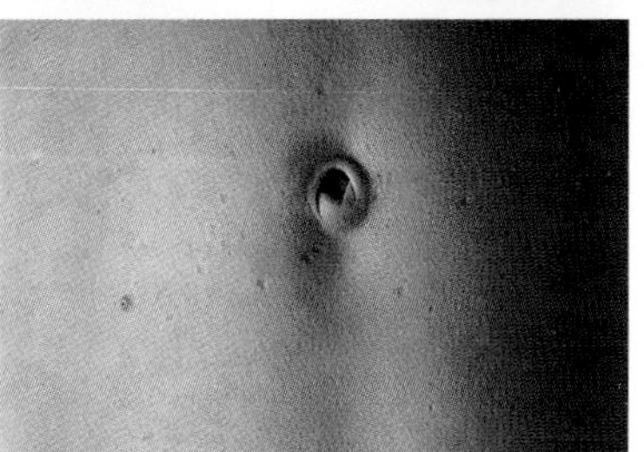

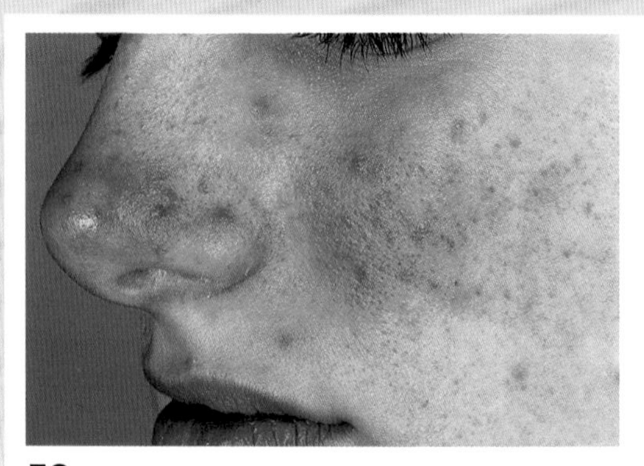

53. This young woman complained of redness and spots on her face associated with increased blushing. She is now 3 months pregnant.

a. What is the diagnosis?
b. How would you treat her?

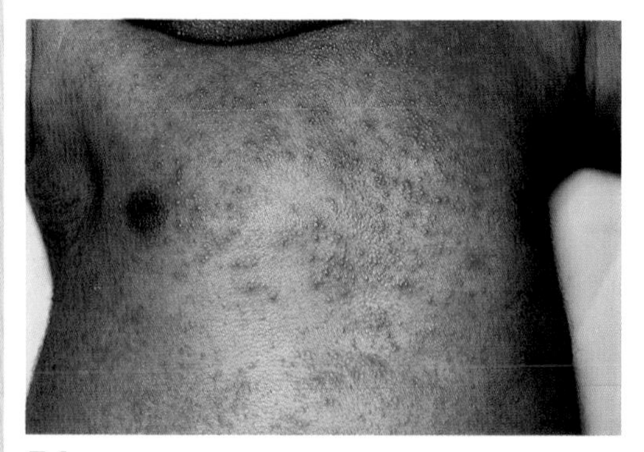

54. This young child presented on a few occasions with this rash. His parents tended to keep him well wrapped up, even in summer.

a. What is the diagnosis?
b. What is the cause?

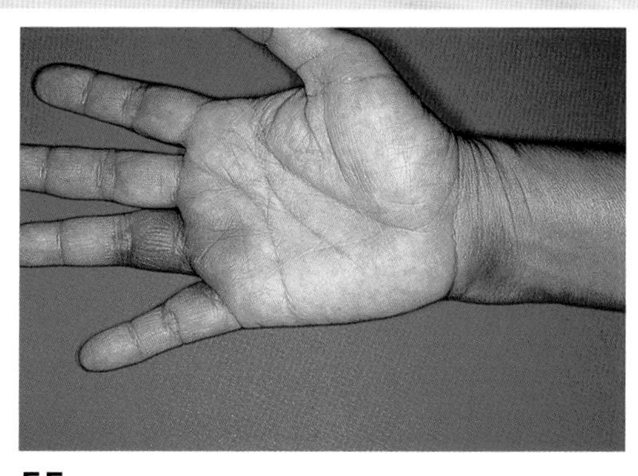

55. This man complained of a recurrent burning eruption affecting his hand, characterized by hyperpigmentation and always affecting the same sites.

a. What is the diagnosis?
b. How might you confirm the diagnosis?
c. List three possible causes.

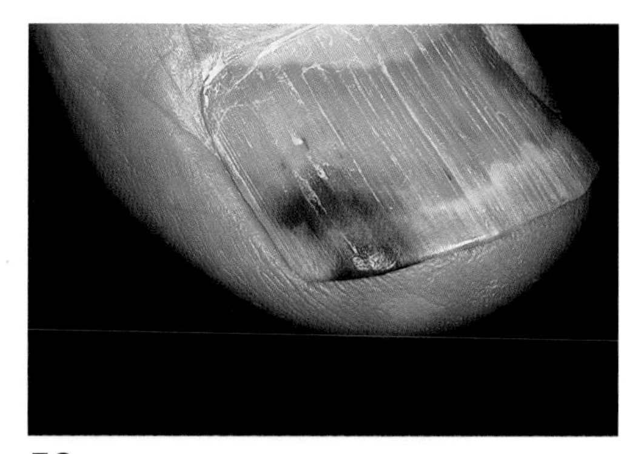

56. A lady had an abnormal nail.

a. What is the cause of this nail's appearance?
b. How would you treat it?

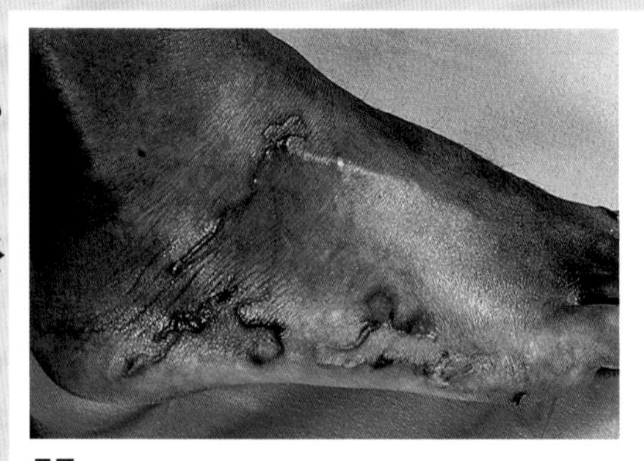

57. This man had just returned from a Caribbean beach holiday with this rash.

a. What is the likely diagnosis?
b. What are the possible causes?
c. How would you treat it?

58. This man had been weeding his garden during the summer whilst wearing shorts.

a. What is the likely diagnosis?
b. List four possible causes.

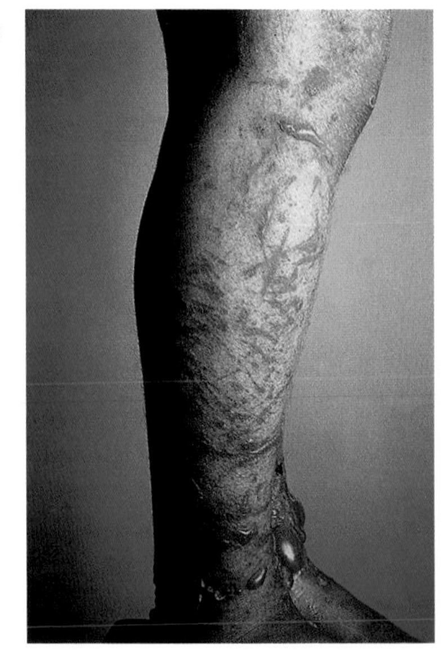

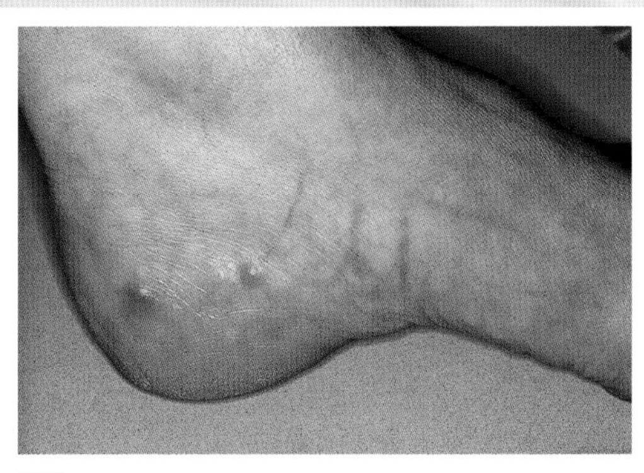

59. This lady presented with painful lesions along the side of her heel, which were only noticeable on standing.

a. What is the diagnosis?
b. What is the presumed patho-aetiology?

60. This patient complained of foot odour and this clinical appearance.

a. What is this condition?
b. How would you treat the patient?

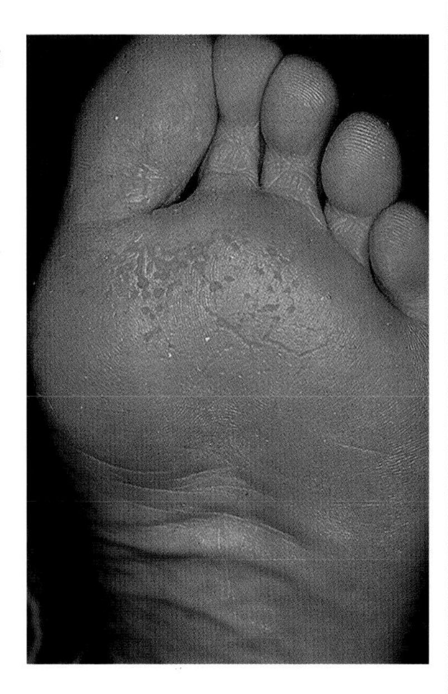

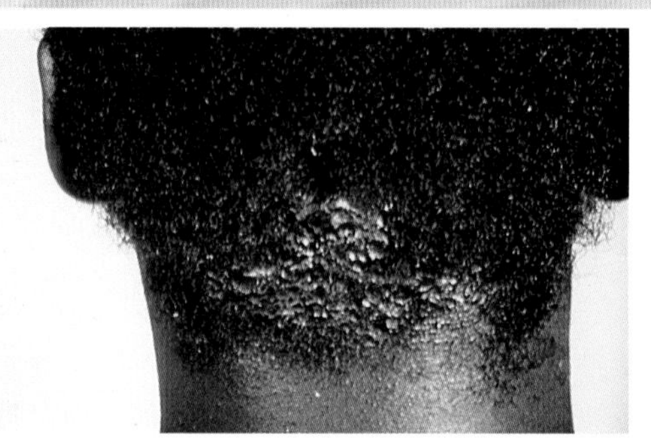

61. This man complained of hair loss and a rash affecting the back of his neck.

a. What is the likely diagnosis?
b. What treatments could be tried?

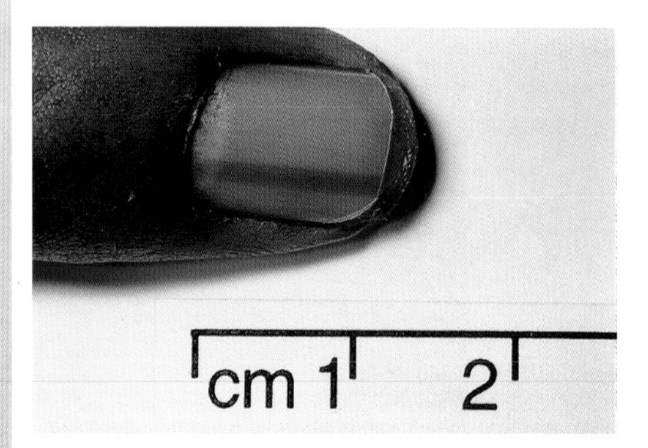

62. This man was concerned about the appearance of his nail.

a. What is the diagnosis?
b. What clinical features help to distinguish this condition?

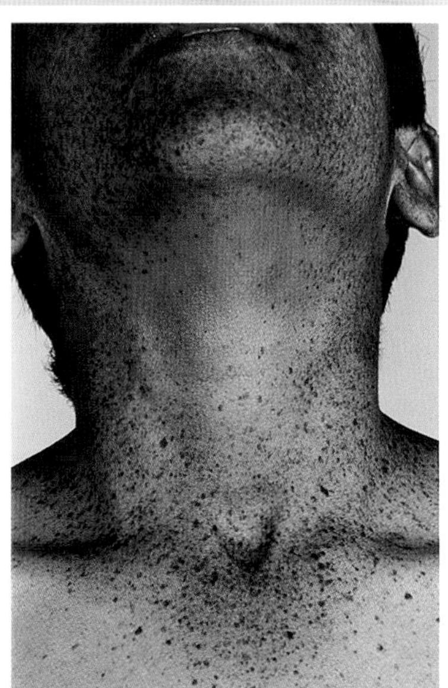

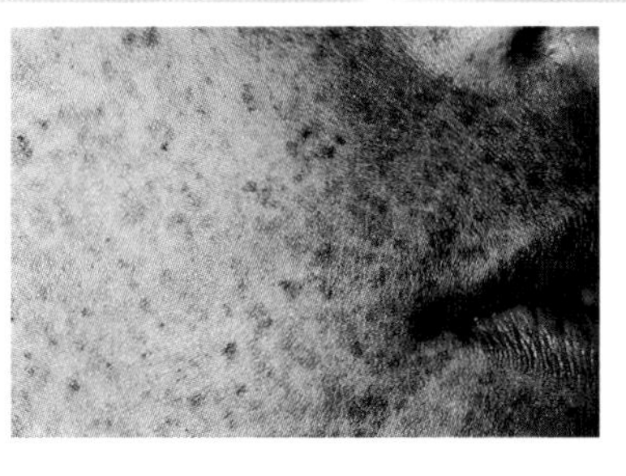

63. This young Asian man started to develop multiple freckles on exposed sites during childhood and has already had two basal cell carcinomas excised.

a. What is the diagnosis?
b. What is the mode of inheritance?
c. How would you confirm the diagnosis?

64. This elderly man developed a symmetrical, asymptomatic, scaly erythematous rash.

a. What is the likely diagnosis?
b. How would you manage this case?

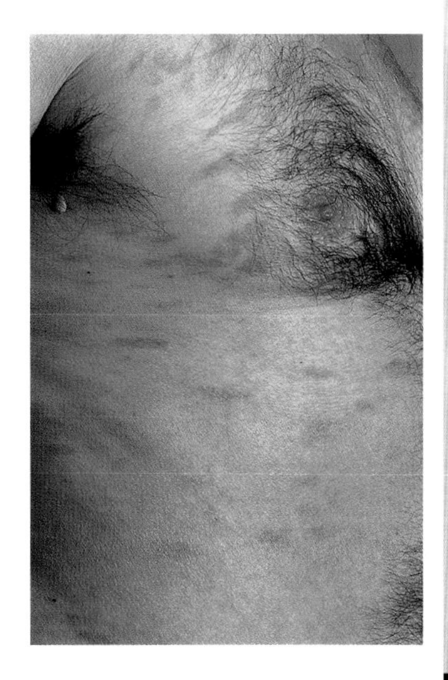

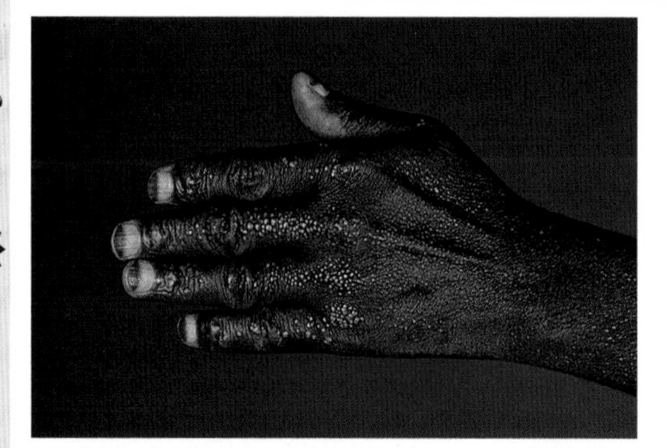

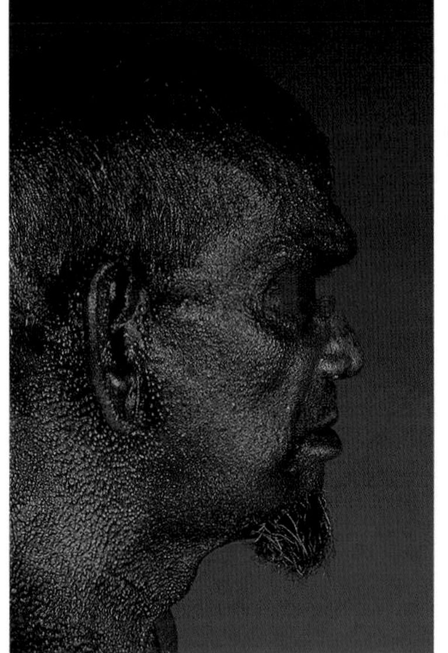

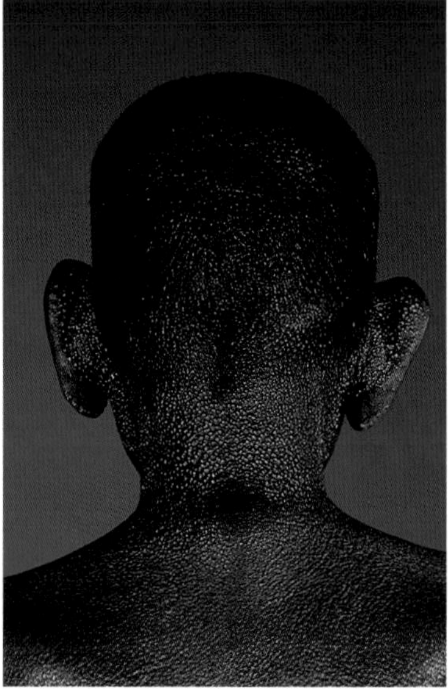

65. This man presented with a widespread pruritic rash predominantly affecting the dorsa of his hands and face, which was associated with dysphagia.

a. What is the likely diagnosis?
b. What blood investigation should be performed?
c. What rare complications can occur?

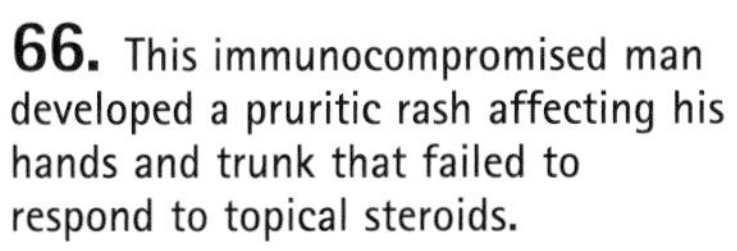

66. This immunocompromised man developed a pruritic rash affecting his hands and trunk that failed to respond to topical steroids.

a. What is the diagnosis?
b. How would you treat this patient?

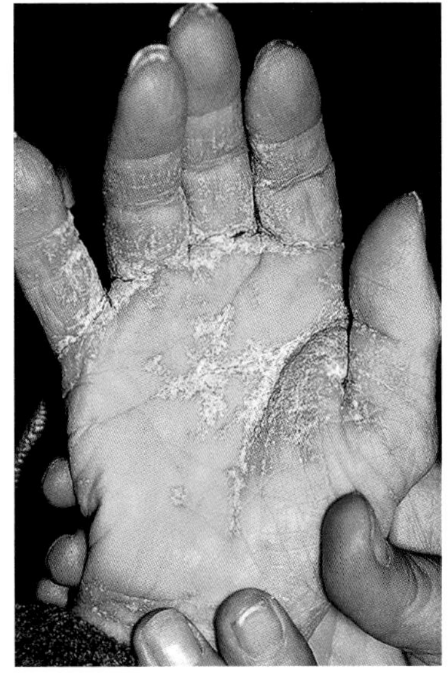

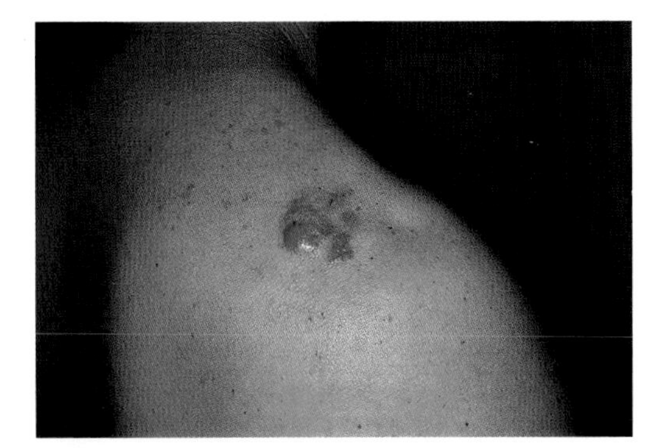

67. This lady developed brownish enlarging nodules on her shoulder.

a. What is the likely diagnosis?
b. What other differential diagnoses should be considered?
c. How should it be managed?

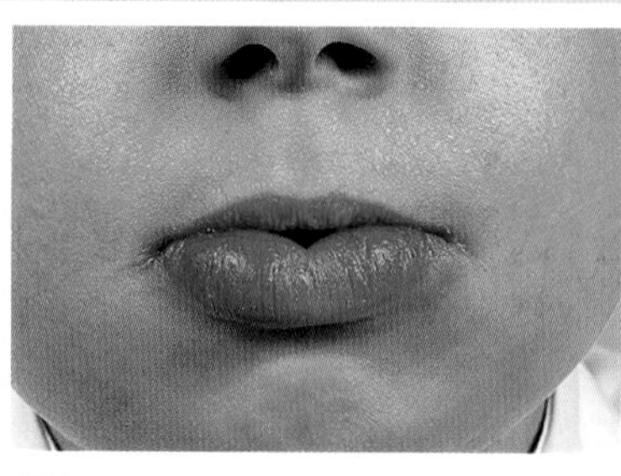

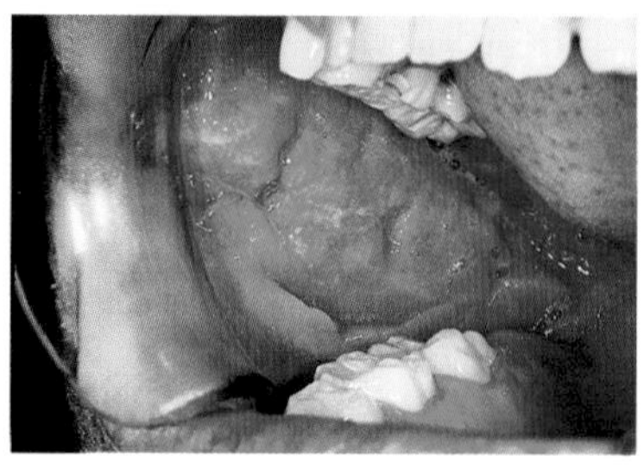

68. This 10-year-old boy had fixed oedema of his lips, with this appearance of the oral cavity and abdominal pain.

a. What is the diagnosis?
b. What would the histology show?
c. What medical treatments have been tried?

69. This man reported a change in his appearance after being started on ciclosporin for psoriasis.

a. What clinical feature is shown in the picture?
b. List three other drugs that have been noted to cause the same effect?

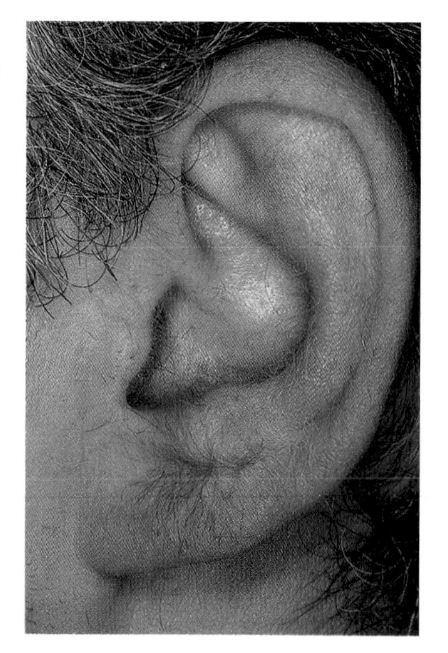

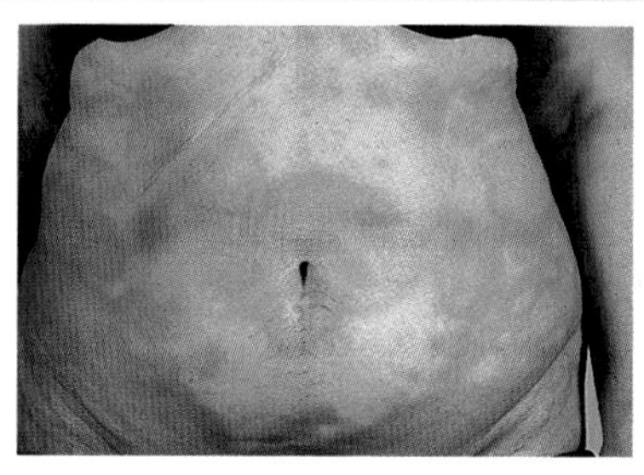

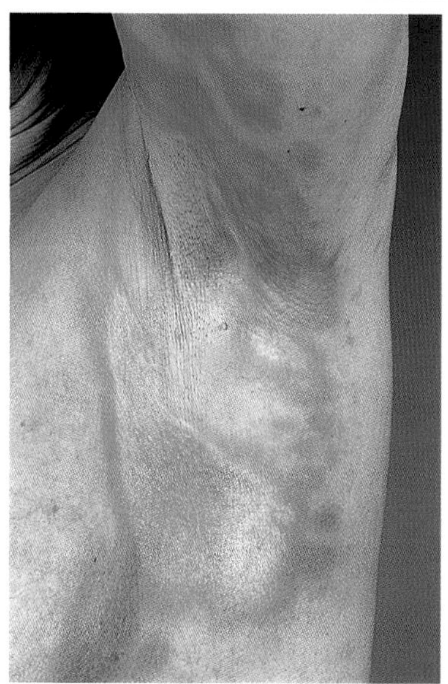

70. This lady presented with a progressive widespread rash.

a. What clinical features are demonstrated in these pictures?
b. What is the diagnosis?
c. What treatments may be tried?

Answers

1. *a.* Peutz–Jegher's syndrome.

b. Autosomal dominant, but up to 40% of cases may be new mutations.

c. Associated with multiple gastrointestinal tract (especially small bowel) polyposis that can cause haemorrhage, obstruction and intussusception, and there is a small risk that the hamartomatous polyps will undergo malignant transformation.

2. *a.*
- café-au-lait macules—a common presenting sign, usually appearing during the first year of life
- axillary freckling
- neurofibromas—may be dome-shaped, pedunculated or plexiform and usually start to develop at puberty and increase in number during adulthood.

b. Neurofibromatosis type 1 (von Recklinghausen's disease). Inheritance is autosomal dominant with 50% of cases representing new mutations.

c. Other clinical findings include Lisch nodules (melanocytic hamartomas of iris), skeletal abnormalities, central nervous system tumours (optic gliomas, astrocytomas, schwannomas) and phaeochromocytomas.

3. *a.*
- ash-leaf macules—hypopigmented macules often appear at birth
- adenoma sebaceum (angiofibromas)—small discrete pink papules mainly affecting the central face and usually not seen until after the age of 5 years
- periungual fibromas—firm, smooth filiform tumours arising from base of nails.

b. Tuberous sclerosis. Autosomal dominant disease with 50–75% spontaneous mutations.

4. *a.*
- hyperextensible joints
- cutis laxa
- atrophic scar.

b. Ehlers–Danlos syndrome—a group of inherited disorders of collagen synthesis with up to 10 phenotypes described.

c. Cutaneous fragility with easy bruising and poor wound healing. Premature onset osteoarthritis of affected joints and life-threatening cerebral and coronary aneurysms in type 4 disease.

5. *a.* Yellow 'pebbly' papules in a reticulate pattern, giving the appearance of 'chicken skin' or 'peau d'orange'.

b. Pseudoxanthoma elasticum. The papules and plaques have a predilection for the lateral neck, antecubital fossae and axillae.

c. Angioid streaks.

d. Patients may be at risk of arterial haemorrhage from the gut or elsewhere, or of vascular occlusion from calcification. Cardiac risk factors should be minimized along with regular ophthalmic review and avoidance of head injury and contact sports.

6. *a.* The ichthyoses (excessive scaling of the skin).

b. Ichthyosis may be inherited as an autosomal dominant trait, sometimes associated with atopy. X-linked ichthyosis is associated with obstetrical and perinatal complications, testicular problems and steroid sulphatase deficiency. Acquired ichthyosis may be due to drugs, various disorders of metabolism, lymphoma, malignancy, immunodeficiency, malabsorption, sarcoidosis and leprosy.

7. *a.* Naevus sebaceous.

b. The naevus may rarely develop a variety of benign and malignant appendageal tumours, basal cell carcinoma or squamous cell carcinoma.

c. Complete excision where feasible, or observation and reporting by the patient of any significant change.

8. *a.* Eczema herpeticum. A widespread disseminated infection of atopic dermatitis by herpes simplex virus.

b. Umbilicated herpetic vesicles that may become haemorrhagic.

9. *a.* Cutaneous atrophy due to thinning of the epidermis and the dermis, showing pronounced telangectasia, striae and steroid purpura.

b. Prolonged and unsupervised prescription and use of potent topical steroids.

10. *a.* Erythema chronicum migrans is the pathognomonic rash occurring early in the course of Lyme borreliosis.

b. A spirochetal infection *(Borrelia burgdorferi)* transmitted to humans by the bite of an infected tick.

c. Oral tetracyclines or amoxicillin.

11. *a.* A mucous digital cyst (myxoid cyst). This is a synovial pseudocyst that most commonly occurs over the distal interphalangeal joints.

b. Distortion of the nail plate and occasionally secondary infection.

c. Excision and repair of the joint capsule offers the best possibility for cure, but drainage of the synovial fluid followed by measures to prevent its reaccumulation can be tried (e.g. intralesional steroid or cryotherapy).

12. *a.* This patient shows features of plain (palm), eruptive (buttock) and nodular (feet) xanthomata. This patient had primary biliary cirrhosis.

b. Fasting lipid profile.

c. Pancreatitis.

13. *a.* Acanthosis nigricans.
b. Underlying malignancy. Cutaneous features that are widespread or involve mucous membranes can predate an underlying malignancy.

14. *a.* Pseudoacanthosis nigricans.
b. Obesity, insulin resistance and other endocrinopathies.

15. *a.* Migratory thrombophlebitis.
b. Erythema gyratum repens, necrolytic migratory erythema, acanthosis nigricans, acquired ichthyosis and generalized pruritus are all well-recognized signs of underlying malignant disease.

16. *a.* Erythema and scaling with a raised border. Skin scrapings are needed for mycological examination.
b. Tinea incognito. The rash initially improves as the steroid suppresses the inflammation, but the infection continues to spread.
c. Topical or systemic antifungal therapy.

17. *a.* Dermatosis papulosa nigra occurs almost exclusively in Afro-Caribbeans.
b. They are benign growths and may be a variant of seborrhoeic keratosis or acrochordon (skin tags). They are best left alone since treatment may leave post-inflammatory hypo- or hyperpigmentation.

18. *a.* Urticaria pigmentosa.
b. Darier's sign.
c. Avoid agents that cause mast cell degranulation. Most children have a good prognosis, with over half of cases resolving by adolescence. Adult patients with urticaria pigmentosa may develop systemic mastocytosis. Systemic antihistamines may be required for symptomatic relief.

19. *a.* The large number of irregularly shaped and pigmented naevi is in keeping with the atypical mole (naevus) syndrome.
b. There is an increased risk of developing a malignant melanoma, especially in patients with a family history of melanoma.
c. Patients need education about sun protection and information about early recognition of suggestive lesions along with regular skin surveillance.

20. *a.*
- cutaneous sarcoidosis
- lupus pernio
- scar sarcoid.

b. Skin biopsy, x-ray of hands and determination of angiotensin converting enzyme (ACE) level for helping to confirm the diagnosis. To help exclude systemic involvement, a chest x-ray, lung function tests, serum calcium and liver function tests, ophthalmic and ear-nose-throat reviews.
c. If hypercalcaemia, eye involvement or significant pulmonary involvement occurred.

21. *a.* Milia and scars (from blisters and skin fragility). Orange-red fluorescence of urine.
b. Porphyria cutanea tarda and haemochromatosis.
c. Porphyria secondary to liver damage from haemochromatosis.
d. Regular venesection to reduce iron stores.

22. *a.* Purpuric and necrotic areas associated with cutaneous vasculitis.
b. Urinalysis and microscopy of urine to exclude renal involvement.
c. A skin biopsy to confirm the diagnosis and to provide clues to the underlying cause. Blood investigations to search for antigens or autoantigens and other organ involvement (e.g. antistreptolysin O [ASO] titre, hepatitis serology, antinuclear factor [ANF], ANCA, rheumatoid factor and other autoantibodies, complement levels, immunoglobulins and acute phase proteins.
d. Bedrest. Elimination or treatment of cause (where possible). Oral steroids with or without other immunosuppressant or anti-inflammatory treatment once infection has been excluded.

23. *a.* Figures show facial and eyelid (heliotrope) erythema with periungual erythema, ragged cuticles and nail fold infarcts.
b. Dermatomyositis. There may also be oedema, photosensitivity, myalgia, muscle tenderness and a proximal myopathy.
c. For diagnosis: skin biopsy, serum creatinine phosphokinase, magnetic resonance imaging, muscle biopsy or electromyography of affected muscle groups. Lung function tests in cases of respiratory muscle involvement. Other investigations would be guided by the clinical history, physical examination or abnormal laboratory tests looking for an underlying malignancy.

24. *a.* Pyoderma gangrenosum.
b. Idiopathic in up to 30% of cases. May be associated with myeloproliferative disease, inflammatory bowel disease, rheumatoid arthritis and chronic active hepatitis.

25. *a.* Perniosis (chilblains).
b. None. Possibility of chilblain, lupus erythematosus and cryoglobulinaemia might be considered.
c. Patients require warm (multilayer) clothing and footwear. Calcium channel blockers (e.g. nifedipine) may be of use in acral idiopathic perniosis.

26. *a.* Livedo reticularis.
b. Cold panniculitis.
c. Livedo reticularis may be idiopathic or secondary—*congenital* (reticulate vascular naevus), *physiological* (cutis marmorata) or associated with *vascular stasis*—but may also be associated with *occlusive vascular disease* (thrombocythaemia, cryoglobulins, cold agglutinins), or *diseases affecting the vessel wall* (arteriosclerosis, polyarteritis nodosa, systemic lupus erythematosus, dermatomyositis, rheumatoid vasculitis).

27. *a.* Scabetic burrow and scabetic nodules.
b. History of others affected (e.g. partners, flatmates, family). Scabies is a disease that flourishes in overcrowded conditions and is spread by close contact.
c. Eczema, urticaria, bullous diseases (e.g. dermatitis herpetiformis, pemphigoid) and lichen planus.

28. *a.* Elastosis perforans serpiginosa.
b. Transepidermal elimination of damaged or abnormal elastic fibres through the skin.
c. 40% of cases are associated with connective tissue disorders, such as pseudo-xanthoma elasticum, Ehlers–Danlos syndrome, Marfan's syndrome, osteogenesis imperfecta and acrogeria. It has also been reported in patients with Down's syndrome and in patients taking penicillamine.
d. Drug-induced pemphigus.

29. *a.* Otitis externa, infected eczematoid dermatitis.
b. Skin swabs for microbiology and patch testing to exclude medicament allergy. Seborrhoeic dermatitis in and around the ear is often secondarily infected. Many cases of chronic otitis externa may develop secondary allergic contact dermatitis to medicaments. Chronic scratching and picking (lichen simplex/neurodermatitis) can often be a perpetuating factor.
c. A combined steroid/antibacterial cream should be used initially with plain steroid preparations subsequently.

30. *a.* An 'inverted champagne bottle' deformity of the lower leg due to lipodermatosclerosis around the ankle, secondary to chronic venous hypertension or venous incompetence.
b. This may be the result of previous deep vein thromboses following one of her earlier operations.

31. *a.* Basal cell carcinoma (rodent ulcer).
b. Solar elastosis and comedones (also associated with chronic sun damage).
c. Excision or superficial radiotherapy to basal cell carcinoma. Examination of other previously sun-exposed sites for evidence of any other skin cancers. Advice regarding sun protection with regular skin surveillance.

32. *a.* Onychomycosis.
b. Nail clippings for fungal microscopy and culture, and examination of skin elsewhere for evidence of tinea infection elsewhere.
c. A 3-month course of oral terbinafine (if dermatophyte) or 3 months of pulsed itraconazole. It may also be appropriate to leave the nails untreated, except for prophylactic antifungal dusting powder, with advice to the patient about using a separate foot towel.

33. *a.* Keloids.
b. May develop following acne (acne keloid), injury or surgery.
c. Keloid scars spread out beyond the site of the original injury.
d. Intralesional steroids, steroid-impregnated tapes, silicone dressings or gels may help if initiated early. Further surgery is usually best avoided.

34. *a.* Chondrodermatitis nodularis helicis.
b. Impaired blood flow to the dermis and underlying cartilage, due to combination of arteriosclerosis and pressure on the ear. May be aggravated by lying preferentially on one side at night and by firm pillows.
c. Excision of nodule (to exclude also basal cell carcinoma, or squamous cell carcinoma) and advice about reducing pressure on the ear.

35. *a.* Cellulitis.
b. Intravenous erythromycin, clindamycin or cephalosporin until pyrexia has resolved. Antibiotics need to cover both group A streptococcus and *Staphylococcus aureus* and should be continued for 14 days.
c. Lymphoedema, previous cellulitis, diabetes, tinea pedis, injuries and ulcers on the lower limbs can predispose to it.
d. Septicaemia, lymphoedema and leg ulceration. Patients with recurrent cellulitis should have prophylactic antibiotics and should wear support stockings (if there is oedema with good arterial circulation).

36. *a.* Podopompholyx.
b. May be constitutional and recurrent (hands and feet) or may be triggered by tinea pedis. Skin scrapings should therefore be taken for fungal microscopy and culture. Rarely, contact dermatitis to footwear may be bullous.

37. *a.* Erythrasma.
b. This is a chronic bacterial infection or intertrigo due to *Corynebacterium minutissimum.*
c. The condition responds to topical fusidic acid and imidazole preparations, and, for widespread infection, oral erythromycin.

38. *a.* A florid morbilliform rash following treatment with ampicillin for sore throat in adolescence or young adults is almost pathognomonic of glandular fever. Differential diagnosis should include post-streptococcal guttate psoriasis, vasculitis and scarlet fever.
b. Examination for general lymphadenopathy with or without splenomegaly and full blood count for atypical lymphocytes or lymphocytosis plus monospot, Paul–Bunnell tests and liver function tests.
c. In 90% of cases, penicillin can be given again later in life without recurrence of a rash. Penicillin must not be given to anyone with a past history of urticaria, angioedema or anaphylactoid reactions to it.

39. *a.* Dental sinus resulting from a dental abscess.
b. Dental x-ray (orthopantomograph).
c. Patient will respond to treatment of the underlying abscess. If only the sinus is excised it will recur.

40. *a.* Nodular prurigo—an intractable and chronic form of prurigo with intense episodic itching resulting in one or multiple nodules, with normal skin interspersed between the lesions. These patients develop a chronic itch-scratch-itch habit.
b. A minority of cases may be associated with underlying haematinic deficiencies or malabsorption.
c. Potent or superpotent topical steroids or intralesional steroids, sedative antihistamines, and bandaging limbs with paste and self-adhesive bandages. Phototherapy may also be helpful.

41. *a.* Bowen's disease or extramammary Paget's disease.
b. Skin biopsy for histology and, in the case of Paget's disease, proctoscopy and sigmoidoscopy to exclude anal or rectal pathology.

42. *a.* Variable pigmentation. The so-called 'red-white-and-blue' sign in a pigmented mole suggests areas of increased vascularity, involution or scarring and dermal pigmentation.
b. Malignant melanoma. Prognosis is determined by depth of invasion.
c. Wide excision (determined by depth) with regular follow-up examinations to check for local recurrence, local lymphadenopathy, development of other suggestive pigmented lesions and systemic spread.

43. *a.* Erythema nodosum (nodular panniculitis if lesions last longer than 3 months).
b. A hypersensitivity response to infectious agents (especially streptococcal), drugs or systemic disease (sarcoidosis, inflammatory bowel disease).
c. Tuberculosis, yersinia, chlamydia, virus (including infectious mononucleosis).
d. Oral contraceptives, sulphonamides, salicylates, iodine and gold salts.

44. *a.* Mucosal (cicatricial) pemphigoid. Inflammatory lesions heal with scarring.
c. May be associated with conjunctivitis, synechiae and keratitis of eyes, hoarseness due to laryngeal involvement, dysphagia from associated oesophageal strictures and sometimes urethral stenosis or labial fusion with anogenital involvement.

45. *a.* Pediculosis capitis or head lice showing the egg cases (nits).
b. Treat the child's scalp with permethrin or malathion scalp application plus regular combing with oil or hair conditioner using a fine-toothed comb. Any secondary infection will need treating. Other children in the

family or friends and classmates will also need to be checked and treated if necessary.

46. *a.* In Behçet's, skin lesions include oral and genital aphthous ulcers, sterile vesiculopustules and pustular vasculitic lesions.
b. Eye symptoms often lag behind mucocutaneous findings and include visual blurring and reduced acuity resulting in blindness if untreated (uveitis, vasculitis and ultimately retinal necrosis). Joint symptoms as a peripheral oligoarticular arthritis may be seen in up to 50% of patients. Headaches, meningismus and even focal neurological signs may occur with central nervous system involvement in severe disease.

47. *a.* Lentigo maligna.
b. Excision, superficial radiotherapy, aggressive cryotherapy and (still experimental) treatment with imiquimod (an extended course).

48. *a.* Melasma (or chloasma when present only around the mouth).
b. Ultraviolet light, hormonal and constitutional factors. Both endogenous female hormones (especially pregnancy) and synthetic oestrogens and progesterone can make the condition worse.
c. Avoid oestrogens and progesterones. Use broad-spectrum sunscreens. Hydroquinone, retinoic acid and glycolic acid peels have also been used.

49. *a.* Necrobiosis lipoidica.
b. Diabetes occurs in up to 60% of cases, and many patients with this condition have impaired glucose tolerance. However, it is rare in the diabetic population (approximately 0.3%).
c. Usually patients are asymptomatic, but the lesions can occasionally ulcerate.

50. *a.* Geographic tongue (benign migratory glossitis).
b. Reassurance. No treatment is necessary since this is a purely physiological phenomenon. Fissured tongue may coexist.

51. *a.* Neuropathic ulcer over a weight-bearing area.
b. Secondary to either diabetic or alcoholic peripheral neuropathy.

52. *a.* Molluscum contagiosum.
b. Lesions can be left to resolve spontaneously or, alternatively, they can be treated with liquid nitrogen after having pre-anaesthetized the skin with topical local anaesthetic.

53. *a.* Acne rosacea.
b. Treatment is difficult during pregnancy, since tetracyclines may be deposited in growing bones and teeth causing staining and occasionally dental hypoplasia; even topical metronidazole would best be avoided. Treatment could be deferred until after completion of breast feeding,

or topical erythromycin or clindamycin could be used. Post partum low-dose oral erythromycin would also be possible.

54. *a.* Miliaria rubra. A large number of uniform nonfollicular papules are seen.
b. A not uncommon rash during the neonatal period, especially in situations of follicular obstruction (e.g. heat and occlusion).

55. *a.* The history is characteristic of a fixed drug eruption.
b. Patch testing with the drug at the site of the lesion may be helpful.
c. The drugs most commonly reported include phenolphthalein in laxatives, sulphonamides and beta-lactam antibiotics.

56. *a.* *Pseudomonas aeruginosa*, which can colonize nail plates that are abnormally lifted up.
b. The abnormal nail should be cut away and the nail bed treated with a topical antiseptic or antibiotic.

57. *a.* Cutaneous larva migrans (creeping eruption).
b. The larvae of dog or cat hookworms (*Ancylostoma caninum* and *A. braziliense*), which migrate through the epidermis.
c. Topical tiabendazole or oral albendazole.

58. *a.* Phytophotodermatitis. This is a phototoxic reaction to plants that contain furocoumarins, causing characteristic linear erythematobullous lesions on exposed sites.
b. Rue, giant hogweed, parsnips (wild and cultivated) and celery.

59. *a.* Piezogenic pedal papules. They may sometimes be painful.
b. Herniation of normal fat into the dermis.

60. *a.* Pitted keratolysis. There are punched out erosions of the stratum corneum caused by coryneform bacteria, often in the presence of hyperhidrosis.
b. Topical antimicrobials (e.g. fucidin or clotrimazole) or systemic erythromycin. Measures to reduce sweating should also be undertaken, including advice on footwear, formaldehyde solution soaks or topical aluminium chloride hexahydrate.

61. *a.* Acne keloidalis nuchae principally occurs in young Afro-Caribbean men. It is a destructive pustulofollicular condition of unknown aetiology that results in keloid nodules and plaques, often devoid of hair.
b. Long-term oral tetracyclines may be helpful for inflammatory pustular lesions. Topical antibiotics may help prevent formation of new lesions. Intralesional steroids may also be used for established keloids.

62. *a.* Linear melanonychia.
b. This is racially common in Afro-Caribbeans and Asians and may affect multiple digits. The pigmentation is usually regular in outline. It is

uncommon in Caucasians, and when it occurs in association with uneven pigmentation or pigmentation of the nail fold (Hutchinson's sign) or surrounding skin, a longitudinal nail biopsy is mandatory.

63. *a.* Xeroderma pigmentosum—a heterogeneous group of conditions that result in premature ageing and skin cancers. It is caused by defective DNA repair following exposure to ultraviolet radiation.
b. Autosomal recessive.
c. Finding of abnormal ultraviolet radiation DNA repair in studies on cultured fibroblasts.

64. *a.* Chronic superficial scaly dermatosis (parapsoriasis en plaque) with characteristic finger-like or digitate processes.
b. Skin biopsy to establish the diagnosis and exclude patch stage mycosis fungoides. Serial skin biopsies if the appearance varies, to exclude progression to mycosis fungoides. Usually no treatment except observation is required, but the condition is responsive to treatment with phototherapy.

65. *a.* Lichen myxoedematosus (papular mucinosis), characterized by waxy firm papules and infiltration of the forehead with prominent supraorbital ridges. On biopsy mucin will be demonstrable in the dermis.
b. Determination of serum immunoglobulins, looking for a paraprotein, usually an immunoglobulin G (IgG) with lambda light chains.
c. Haematological malignancies, including myeloma or Waldenström's macroglobulinaemia.

66. *a.* Norwegian scabies (crusted scabies). This occurs with extensive infestation of the scabies mite, often in immunocompromised or institutionalized patients.
b. Apart from the usual topical treatments, including malathion and permethrin, and along with careful tracing and treatment of patient's contacts, consider ivermectin (not currently licensed for scabies).

67. *a.* Dermatofibrosarcoma protuberans—a low-grade malignant soft tissue tumour of fibroblasts.
b. Keloids, dermatofibromas.
c. They rarely metastasize but have an infiltrating growth pattern that often extends beyond the clinical margins. Wide excision, possibly involving Moh's surgery, should be performed.

68. *a.* Oral Crohn's disease.
b. Non-caseating granulomas and oedema.
c. Intralesional and systemic steroids for oral involvement and consideration of other immunosuppressants for other bowel involvement.

69. *a.* Drug-induced hypertrichosis.
b. Corticosteroids, diazoxide and penicillamine.

70. *a.* Widespread large hypopigmented plaques with shiny surfaces, some surrounded by an erythematous margin.
b. Generalized morphoea. It is not associated with systemic disturbance.
c. Generalized morphoea can last for years, although some spontaneous improvement can be expected. There is no specific treatment, but systemic steroids, penicillamine, high-dose antimalarials and high-dose UVA have all been tried.

Index

A

B

C

D

E

F

G

H

I

O

P